## Advanced Acclaim for
### *If Your Adolescent Has Depression or Bipolar Disorder*

"A truly essential resource for parents of adolescents with depression or bipolar disorder. Clearly written, practical, and thoroughly up-to-date, this book focuses on the specific challenges of getting the best treatment for teens. Read this book, not just to know, but to know how."

—Kate Pravera, Ph.D., Executive Director,
Child and Adolescent Bipolar Foundation

"This is a wonderful, understandable, science-based resource for parents trying to understand and help their teenagers who are suffering much more than the usual turmoil of adolescence. It speaks both to the origins and treatments of adolescent depression, and helps parents understand what they can and can't do to help their children."

—Alan I. Leshner, MD, Chief Executive Officer,
American Association for the Advancement of Science,
Executive Publisher, *Science*

"An extremely helpful guide for parents feeling powerless, afraid, lost, or paralyzed. In easy to understand language, it covers difficult topics such as suicide, involuntary hospitalization, explosive situations, and school bullying. This guide explains how parents can help their child while taking care of themselves."

—Lydia Lewis, President,
Depression and Bipolar Support Alliance

"This book provides a clear, intelligent explanation of what depression and bipolar disorder are. And it offers many directions and resources to help parents and teens cope with these serious but treatable illnesses. For those of us in families with depression or bipolar disorder—that is, almost all of us—this book delivers three crucial things: knowledge, help, and hope."

—Paul Raeburn, Author of
*Acquainted with the Night: A Parent's Quest to Understand
Depression and Bipolar Disorder in His Children*

"This book by Evans and Andrews . . . is concise and easy to read, yet amazingly comprehensive and filled with practical, clinically and scientifically sound information. Since there is no other book like this one available, it fills an important, unmet need for parents. . . . Clinicians will also find it very helpful as a highly informative book, either to give or recommend to the parents of younger patients that they are treating for mood disorders."

—Lewis L. Judd, M.D.
Mary Gilman Marston Professor, and Chair,
Department of Psychiatry, University of California, San Diego

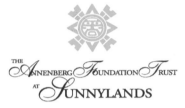

The Annenberg Foundation Trust at Sunnylands'
Adolescent Mental Health Initiative

Patrick Jamieson, PhD, *series editor*

Other books in the series

*If Your Adolescent Has an Eating Disorder (Fall 2005)*
B. Timothy Walsh, MD, and V. L. Cameron

*If Your Adolescent Has an Anxiety Disorder (2006)*
Edna B. Foa, PhD, and Linda Wasmer Andrews

*If Your Adolescent Has Schizophrenia (2006)*
Raquel E. Gur, MD, PhD, and Ann Braden Johnson, PhD

# If Your Adolescent Has Depression or Bipolar Disorder

*An Essential Resource for Parents*

Dwight L. Evans, MD, and Linda Wasmer Andrews

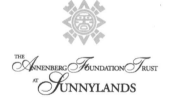

The Annenberg Foundation Trust at Sunnylands'
Adolescent Mental Health Initiative

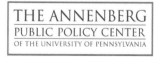

## OXFORD
### UNIVERSITY PRESS

2005

# OXFORD
UNIVERSITY PRESS

Oxford University Press, Inc., publishes works that
further Oxford University's objective of excellence
in research, scholarship, and education.

The Annenberg Foundation Trust at Sunnylands
The Annenberg Public Policy Center of the University of Pennsylvania
Oxford University Press

Oxford   New York
Auckland   Cape Town   Dar es Salaam   Hong Kong   Karachi
Kuala Lumpur   Madrid   Melbourne   Mexico City   Nairobi
New Delhi   Shanghai   Taipei   Toronto

With offices in
Argentina   Austria   Brazil   Chile   Czech Republic   France   Greece
Guatemala   Hungary   Italy   Japan   Poland   Portugal   Singapore
South Korea   Switzerland   Thailand   Turkey   Ukraine   Vietnam

Published by Oxford University Press, Inc.
198 Madison Avenue, New York, New York 10016
www.oup.com

Library of Congress Cataloging-in-Publication Data
Evans, Dwight L.
If your adolescent has depression or bipolar disorder : an essential resource for parents /
by Dwight L. Evans and Linda Wasmer Andrews.
  p.   cm. — (Adolescent mental health initiative)
ISBN-10: 0-19-518209-X (cloth)   ISBN-13: 978-0-19-518209-5 (cloth-13)
ISBN-10: 0-19-518210-3 (pbk)     ISBN-13: 978-0-19-518210-1 (pbk-13)
1. Depression in adolescence—Popular works.
2. Manic-depressive illness in adolescence—Popular works.
3. Parenting.
I. Andrews, Linda Wasmer. II. Title. III. Series.
RJ506.D4E93 2005
618.92'8527—dc22   2004028088

9 8 7 6 5 4 3 2
Printed in the United States of America on acid-free paper

# Contents

# Foreword

The Adolescent Mental Health Initiative (AMHI) was created by The Annenberg Foundation Trust at Sunnylands to share with mental health professionals, parents, and adolescents the advances in treatment and prevention now available to adolescents with mental health disorders. The Initiative was made possible by the generosity and vision of Ambassadors Walter and Leonore Annenberg, and the project was administered through the Annenberg Public Policy Center of the University of Pennsylvania in partnership with the Oxford University Press.

The Initiative began in 2003 with the convening, in Philadelphia and New York, of seven scholarly commissions made up of over 150 leading psychiatrists and psychologists from around the country. Chaired by Drs. Edna B. Foa, Dwight L. Evans, B. Timothy Walsh, Martin E.P. Seligman, Raquel E. Gur, Charles P. O'Brien, and Herbert Hendin, these commissions were tasked with assessing the state of scientific research on the prevalent mental disorders whose onset occurs predominantly between the ages of 10 and 22. Their collective findings now appear in a book for mental health professionals and policy makers titled *Treating and Preventing Adolescent Mental Health Disorders*

(2005). As the first product of the Initiative, that book also identified a research agenda that would best advance our ability to prevent and treat these disorders, among them anxiety disorders, depression and bipolar disorder, eating disorders, substance abuse, and schizophrenia.

The second prong of the Initiative's three-part effort is a series of books, including this one, that are designed primarily for parents of adolescents with a specific mental health disorder. Drawing their scientific information largely from the AMHI professional volume, these "parent books" present each relevant commission's findings in an accessible way and in a voice that we believe will be both familiar and reassuring to parents and families of an adolescent-in-need. In addition, this series, which will be followed by another targeted for adolescent readers themselves, combines medical science with the practical wisdom of parents who have faced these illnesses in their own children.

The third part of the Sunnylands Adolescent Mental Health Initiative consists of two websites. The first, www.CopeCare Deal.org, addresses teens. The second, www.oup.com/us/teenmentalhealth, provides updates to the medical community on matters discussed in *Treating and Preventing Adolescent Mental Health Disorders*, the AMHI professional book.

We hope that you find this volume, as one of the fruits of the Initiative, to be helpful and enlightening.

Patrick Jamieson, Ph.D.
*Series Editor*
*Adolescent Risk Communication Institute*
*Annenberg Public Policy Center*
*University of Pennsylvania*
*Philadelphia, PA*

# If Your Adolescent Has Depression or Bipolar Disorder

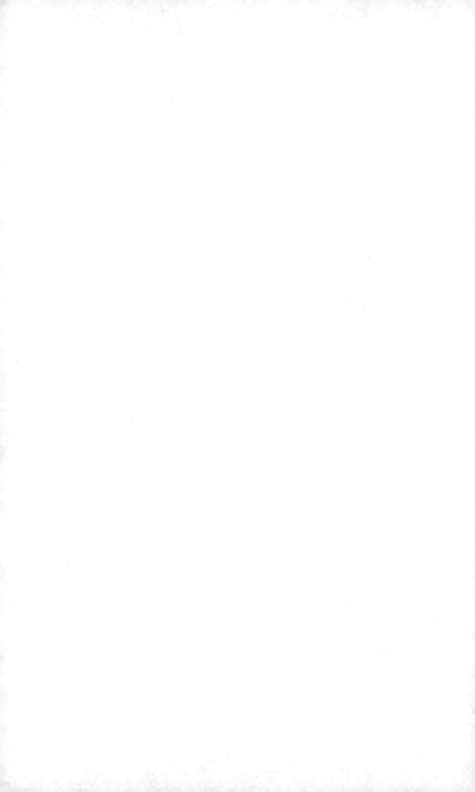

## Chapter One

# Introduction: More Than Ordinary Moodiness

Adolescence is a time of growth and maturation, and change is an inevitable part of that process. For some parents, though, there comes a moment of truth when they realize that their teenagers are experiencing something more than the ordinary ups and downs:

"One day, she trotted off to school and had a mini-breakdown at lunch. She started crying and couldn't stop. She got so upset that the school called me to come pick her up." —Parent of a 14-year-old girl

"He became the life of the party—kind of like Jim Carrey in a movie. But the warning bells went off when he started running five miles at 2:00 in the morning." —Parent of a 15-year-old boy

"She was screaming and screaming, totally out of control. She weighed 90 pounds, she was barefoot—and she kicked a hole about 18 inches in diameter in the wall of her bedroom." —Parent of a 17-year-old girl

"A friend told me he had been cutting on himself with a knife, but in places where I couldn't see, like on his legs. He always wore long pants, so I knew it wasn't to get attention." —Parent of a 15-year-old boy

"In the space of a few hours, the guidance counselor, the English teacher, and the music teacher all called to say they were afraid she was considering taking her own life." —Parent of a 16-year-old girl

For other parents, the realization that something is wrong dawns more gradually, but is no less disturbing once it hits. Perhaps your formerly sunny child has stopped smiling and seems to have a dark cloud always hanging over his or her head. Or perhaps your child who once seemed merely active now seems to be moving through life with the unstoppable energy and destructive force of a tornado. Of course, there are many possible explanations for a drastic change in attitude and behavior. However, for as many as one-quarter of adolescents, the changes may be due, at least in part, to a mood disorder.

*. . . your formerly sunny child has stopped smiling . . .*

## Depths of Depression, Highs of Mania

Scientifically speaking, a mood is a pervasive emotion that colors a person's whole view of the world. As you might expect, a mood disorder leads to major disturbances in mood. Such disorders can be broken down into two main categories: depression and bipolar disorder. Depression, as the term is used here, is more than just an occasional case of the blues or the blahs. Instead, it's a feeling of being sad, hopeless, apathetic, or down in the dumps that lasts for at least a couple of weeks and interferes with a person's life at home, school, or work.

Bipolar disorder—once called manic depression—is characterized by an overly high mood, called mania, that alternates with depression. A teenager in the grips of mania may seem very irritable or excessively silly. Or the teen may seem to be operating at warp speed—doing six things at once, talking too much or too fast, going for days with little sleep, or showing signs of racing thoughts or exaggerated beliefs. In young people with bipolar disorder, depression often appears first, only to be followed later by mania. The result can be a wild emotional ride, as the teen's rollercoaster moods fluctuate between extreme lows and extreme highs.

During a bout of depression or mania, teenagers can wreak havoc on the lives of those around them. They may spark conflict at home or create disruptions in the classroom. Their problems—ranging from withdrawal and suicidal behavior to substance abuse and violent outbursts—can monopolize so much of your time and energy that you have little left for your spouse and other children, let alone for yourself. You may feel as if you're constantly on high alert or walking on eggshells in your own home. And as if that weren't stressful enough, you may find yourself fielding unhappy calls from the school principal, parents of your teen's friends, or even the police.

*You may feel as if you're constantly on high alert . . .*

Yet as difficult as the situation may be for you, it's twice as tough for your teen. For a parent, the hardest thing of all may be watching a child sink into despair or self-destructive behavior, and feeling helpless to prevent the downward slide. The good news is that help is out there, if you just know where to look. As alone and frightened as you may feel at times, there are millions of other parents going through much the same thing and feeling much the same way. And as overwhelming and confusing as all this may be, we now know more about teen depression and bipolar disorder than ever before, and we're adding to that knowledge each day.

How can you tell if your teenager is just moody or something more? The only way to know for sure is to have your teen evaluated by a qualified mental health professional. No book can take the place of professional diagnosis and treatment. What this book *can* do, however, is answer some of the pressing questions that may arise if your adolescent is having severe mood swings or if your teen has already been diagnosed with depression or bipolar disorder. For example,

- Are my teenager's mood swings normal?
- If my teen has a mood disorder, is it my fault?
- Where can I find good care for my child?
- How safe and effective are the treatment options?
- Will insurance pay for these treatments?
- What are the warning signs of suicide?
- Will our family life always seem chaotic?
- How can I help my child succeed at school?
- What does the future hold for my child?
- Where can I find further support and education?

The most important step you can take to help your teen is to empower yourself. As the cliché goes, knowledge is power. The more you know, the better equipped you'll be to ask crucial questions, make informed decisions, and, when necessary, advocate for additional services with your insurance company or school system. As a result, the greater your teenager's chances will be of getting effective treatment and an appropriate education. You can make the critical difference.

*You can make the critical difference.*

## Using This Book

There may be times when you need fast answers to a question about your teen's current situation, and we've tried to organize the book in a way that makes it easy to find depression- or bipolar-specific information. When time allows, however, we suggest that you read the entire book, since there is considerable overlap between the two conditions. Studies have found that a substantial minority of adolescents with depression go on to develop bipolar disorder within 5 years. Conversely, most adolescents with bipolar disorder have periods of depression that alternate or coincide with periods of mania.

The lead author of this book is a psychiatrist with several hundred publications to his name on the biological, psychological, and social factors associated with mood disorders. He is a professor of psychiatry, medicine, and neuroscience as well as chairman of the psychiatry department at the University of Pennsylvania School of Medicine. In 2003, he served as chair of a professional Commission on Adolescent Depression and Bipolar Disorder, part of the Adolescent Mental Health Initiative spearheaded by the Annenberg Foundation Trust at Sunnylands; it is from the report of that commission that this book draws much of its scientific information. And in 2005, he became president of the American Foundation for Suicide Prevention. Among the honors he has received are the 1997 Gerald L. Klerman Lifetime Research Award from the National Depressive and Manic Depressive Association (now the Depression and Bipolar Support Alliance) and the 2004 Award for Research in Mood Disorders from the American College of Psychiatrists. Along with a lifetime commitment to improving the lives of patients and families, he brings a wealth of mental health experience and expertise to this project. The result is a book that reflects the latest state of the science on the diagnosis, treatment, management, and prevention of teen mood disorders. In this regard, we'd like to thank Moira A. Rynn, MD, assistant professor of psychiatry and medical director of the Mood and Anxiety Disorders Section at the University of Pennsylvania School of

Medicine, for her assistance in reviewing and providing feedback on the scientific dimensions of the book.

The coauthor of this book is a journalist who has specialized in mental health issues for two decades. Her most important role on this project was to interview parents from across the country and bring their voices to these pages. The parents she talked and e-mailed with know what it's like to raise an adolescent with depression or bipolar disorder because they've all been there themselves. These mothers and fathers were extremely generous about sharing their insights, and the book is filled with their parent-tested advice and practical support. To protect the privacy of the parents and their families, names have been changed. Otherwise, the stories are true, and we think you'll find the down-to-earth wisdom and hands-on suggestions of these experienced parents especially helpful.

*Chapter Two*

# Understanding the Disorders:
# What They Are, What to Expect

---

A s the parent of an adolescent with depression or bipolar disorder, you may be feeling confused, concerned, and convinced that you're the only one who has ever tried to cope with such powerful mood swings in a child. In truth, however, you are far from alone. Laurel is just one of the many, many parents who have stood in your shoes:

*. . . you are far from alone.*

"Looking back, I probably wasn't aware when Carly first started having problems," Laurel recalls. "I noticed that she had started acting out and being belligerent and running around with a different crowd than usual. But I didn't think too much of it. Then she tried to commit suicide."

If Laurel missed some crucial early warning signs, it was understandable. After years of working hard as a single mother to provide a stable, comfortable home for her three children, Laurel had recently suffered some serious setbacks. Just months earlier, Laurel had married again, only to find that her new husband had a drinking problem. Before long, he was involved in a drunken driving accident that landed him in jail. Around the same time, Laurel discovered that she had cervical cancer. The stress in her life had suddenly shot up to astronomical levels, and the children, all teenagers by this point, weren't making things any easier. In the midst of the turmoil, Laurel failed to notice that 14-year-old Carly's own distress had gradually deepened into something much darker.

Then the morning after Laurel returned home from having cancer surgery, something unusual happened: Carly failed to get ready for school on time. "This child had never been late for school before," Laurel says. "I told her to hurry up. I was going to take her sister to school, and then come back for her. It's a four-block drive up and back—probably 3 minutes that I was gone. When I got home, I found Carly on the floor." She had taken two bottles of Laurel's prescription pills—an antidepressant and a sleep aid—as well as some over-the-counter medications.

Laurel was able to get her daughter to the emergency room quickly, and the physical aftereffects of the overdose were minimal. The depression was not so easy to shake, however. After a brief psychiatric hospitalization, Carly returned home, but she continued to see a psychiatrist and take medication, and the family began going to counseling. Since she was still too ill to attend school, Carly was put on homebound instruction. A teacher visited once a week, and her mother helped with her lessons between visits. Laurel revamped her own schedule, too. As a music teacher who taught in her home, "I thought I was available, because I was here all the time," she says. "But I realized that I was always with a student. So I dropped a lot of students, and I rearranged my schedule so that I had 30 minutes of uninterrupted time with the girls every afternoon." Finally, Laurel decided to file for divorce and try to get her personal life back on a steady footing.

The next fall, Carly was able to return to high school, thanks largely to a caring school counselor who helped her through the transition. "She bounced back and graduated with honors," Laurel says. Her first year of college, Carly chose a school that was more than 4 hours away from home. "Around February of her first year there, she became depressed again," says Laurel. "She said it wasn't as bad as before and she didn't want counseling, but she did start taking medication. Between my mother and me, we called her at least once or twice a day, and I talked to her on Instant Messenger a lot." Carly made it through the semester with good grades, and, at this writing, was preparing for her second year away.

"I was absolutely paralyzed with fear . . ."

Recalling the suicide attempt, Laurel says, "I was just so scared. I was absolutely paralyzed with fear at first. But I remember thinking, I'll put my head down and push through this—always prioritizing the list, always making sure the kids are in the right place on the list. Because no matter what comes on you, you just do what you have to do, especially if you're a parent."

You may recognize a little of yourself in Laurel, even if the details of your own story are quite different. One thing the two of you undoubtedly have in common is a strong desire to help your teen win the struggle against dark or self-destructive moods. The first step is learning more about the symptoms, causes, and consequences of depression and bipolar disorder.

## Depression: Characteristics, Causes, and Risk Factors; Other Conditions; Outlook for the Future

Everyone feels a little down now and then, and your teenager is no exception. However, true depression is much more than just a passing blue mood. It's an illness that affects the brain and body at every level—emotionally, mentally, physically, and behaviorally. The operative word here is "illness." Depression is not a character flaw or a reflection on your skills as a parent. Instead, it's every bit as much a "real" disease as asthma or diabetes. You wouldn't ask a child with asthma to just think positively the next time he's having trouble breathing or one with diabetes to simply hope for the best the next time her blood sugar levels start to shoot through the roof. Instead, you would surely try to provide the best possible professional treatment coupled with lots of parental support. The same approach applies equally well to depression.

Without treatment, depression can last for weeks, months, or even years. It can affect every facet of your teenager's life, including home and school routine as well as relationships with family and friends. Depression can also contribute to academic failure, substance abuse, or suicidal thoughts. The mental anguish for your teen—and the strain on you and your family as you watch this suffering—can exact a harsh toll on everyone.

It doesn't have to be this way. Most people with depression—even those with severe symptoms—can be helped to feel better with proper treatment. In fact, it's estimated that 80% to 90% of all cases of depression can be treated successfully, although it sometimes may take a few tries to find the best treatment for a particular individual. Unfortunately, adequate treatment seems to be more the exception than the rule, especially when it comes to children and adolescents. A conference held by the U.S. Surgeon General in 2000 found that fewer than 1 in 5 young people with a mental disorder serious enough to cause some impairment actually received the treatment he or she needed. This disheartening statistic just underscores the crucial role that parents play. It's a good bet that most of those fortunate 20% had someone actively seeking treatment for them and speaking up on their behalf.

> . . . it sometimes may take a few tries to find the best treatment for a particular individual.

### What Is Major Depression?

The *DSM-IV-TR* (short for *Diagnostic and Statistical Manual of Mental Disorders*, Fourth Edition, Text Revision) is a manual that mental health professionals use for diagnosing all kinds of mental illnesses. This manual defines major depression as essentially either being depressed or irritable nearly all the time, or losing interest or enjoyment in almost everything. These feelings last for at least 2 weeks and are associated with other symptoms, such as a change in eating or sleeping habits, lack of energy, feelings of worthlessness, trouble with concentration, or thoughts of suicide.

# Major Depression

Below are the *DSM-IV-TR* criteria for major depression in adolescents:

1. At least one of the following symptoms must occur most of the day, nearly every day, for 2 weeks or longer.

    a. A depressed mood (for example, feelings of sadness or emptiness); in adolescents, the mood may be irritable instead

    b. A marked loss of interest or pleasure in all or most of the things that the person once enjoyed

2. At least three or four of the following symptoms must occur during the same 2-week period. (The total number of symptoms from this group and the previous one should add up to five or more.) The symptoms should represent a change from the person's usual functioning.

    a. Significant weight loss without dieting, excessive weight gain, or a decrease or increase in appetite

    b. Insomnia or oversleeping

    c. Behavior that seems either overly keyed up or unnaturally slowed down

    d. Constant fatigue or lack of energy

    e. Feelings of worthlessness or inappropriate guilt

    f. Reduced ability to concentrate, think clearly, or make decisions

    g. Recurrent thoughts of death or suicide

3. The symptoms cause significant distress or impairment at home, school, or work.

4. The symptoms are not due to the direct physiological effects of alcohol or drug abuse, a general medical condition, or the side effects of a medication.

---

Adapted from American Psychiatric Association, *Diagnostic and Statistical Manual of Mental Disorders* (4th ed., text revision, p. 356). Washington, DC: American Psychiatric Association, 2000.

## Can Major Depression Take Different Forms?

While there are common symptoms that characterize the illness, no two individuals experience depression in exactly the same way.

*. . . no two individuals experience depression in exactly the same way.*

In addition to garden-variety major depression, psychiatrists have identified several subtypes of the disorder:

- Chronic—All the symptoms of major depression have been present continuously for at least 2 years.
- Catatonic—Although all the criteria for major depression are met, the most prominent symptoms involve behavior that seems either slowed down or keyed up. These symptoms may include physical immobility, stupor, purposeless overactivity, extreme negativism, refusal to speak, peculiar mannerisms, grimacing, parrot-like repetition of someone else's words, or mimicking of another's movements.
- Melancholic—The dominant feature is a near-complete lack of interest or pleasure in almost all activities. The person's mood never brightens, even temporarily, when something good happens. Other symptoms may include depression that is worse in the morning, waking up too early, behavior that seems either slowed down or keyed up, significant weight loss, lack of appetite, or inappropriate guilt.
- Psychotic—In addition to other symptoms of severe depression, the person may have delusions. These are bizarre beliefs that are out of touch with reality, such as the belief that one's thoughts can be heard by others. Or the person may have hallucinations. These are sensory perceptions of things that aren't really there, such as hearing voices.

- Atypical—This type of depression is not as uncommon as its name might imply, especially in young people. The hallmark is the ability to cheer up when something good happens. However, the person then sinks back into depression as soon as the positive event has passed. Other symptoms may include significant weight gain, increase in appetite, oversleeping, a weighed-down feeling in the arms or legs, or a longtime pattern of hypersensitivity to personal rejection.
- Seasonal (also known as seasonal affective disorder, or SAD)—The symptoms of depression start and stop around the same time each year. Typically, they begin in fall or winter and subside in spring. The onset seems to be linked directly to the change of season—in particular, reduced exposure to sunlight in winter—rather than the start of school. Symptoms may include lack of energy, oversleeping, overeating, weight gain, and a craving for sugary or starchy foods.
- Postpartum—The symptoms of depression begin within 4 weeks of giving birth. The depression is more severe, prolonged, and disabling than the ordinary baby blues that many new mothers have for a few days. Postpartum depression can occur in teenage girls who have babies just as it does in older women.

**What Is Dysthymia?**

A second type of depression is called dysthymia. For the most part, dysthymia produces the same symptoms as major depression, although they are less severe. But while the symptoms are milder, they can still cause a lot of misery, because they hang around for at least a year. It's somewhat like the difference between mild, chronic allergies and a bad case of the flu. The

## Dysthymia

Below are the *DSM-IV-TR* criteria for dysthymia in adolescents:

1. A depressed or irritable mood most of the day, more days than not, for 12 months or longer.
2. At least two of the following symptoms must occur during the same period. The person is never symptom-free for more than 2 months at a time.
   a. Overeating or poor appetite
   b. Insomnia or oversleeping
   c. Constant fatigue or lack of energy
   d. Low self-esteem
   e. Trouble concentrating or making decisions
   f. Feelings of hopelessness
3. The symptoms cause significant distress or impairment at home, school, or work.
4. The symptoms are not due to the direct physiological effects of alcohol or drug abuse, a general medical condition, or the side effects of a medication.

---

Adapted from American Psychiatric Association, *Diagnostic and Statistical Manual of Mental Disorders* (4th ed., text revision, pp. 380–381). Washington, DC: American Psychiatric Association, 2000.

flu symptoms are more severe, but the allergy symptoms can still have a significant effect on a person's quality of life.

### What Warning Signs Should You Watch For?

Depression is an insidious disease. It may start out as a relatively mild case of the blues or anxiety that worsens over time. Often, the transition to full-blown depression is so slow and gradual that parents miss the warning signs until something drastic happens. As with any other illness, however, the earlier depression is professionally diagnosed and treated, the sooner the suffering can be relieved, and the better the outcome is likely to be. Watch for these red flags in your teenager:

- Decreased interest in friends and activities
- Difficulty concentrating
- A drop in grades or frequent absences from school
- Complaints of tiredness or boredom
- Vague physical symptoms, such as unexplained aches and pains
- Changes in sleep patterns, such as insomnia or oversleeping
- Increased crankiness, hostility, or anger
- Outbursts of shouting or crying
- Reckless behavior
- Alcohol or drug abuse
- Trouble getting along with others
- Social withdrawal
- Hypersensitivity to rejection or failure
- Self-injurious behavior or talk of suicide

**How Is Depression Diagnosed?**

Life would be simpler if there were a blood test or even a sophisticated brain scan that could definitely diagnose depression. Unfortunately, there isn't. To make a formal diagnosis of major depression or dysthymia, a mental health professional or physician must evaluate a person's symptoms and then try to decide whether they meet the criteria laid out in the *DSM-IV-TR*. In adults, most of the information about history and current symptoms is gleaned from talking to the patients themselves. In adolescents, however, not only the young patients but also the parents are key sources of information. Parents know their children's life history better than anyone else does. Parental input is also invaluable because the teenagers themselves may have trouble expressing their true feelings, lack insight into them, or be uncooperative at first.

*Parents know their children's life history better than anyone else does.*

When meeting with your child's mental health care provider for the first time, come prepared to answer questions about the behaviors that concern you, including when they started, how often they occur, how long they last, and how severe they seem. Other potential sources of information, depending on the situation, may include teachers, school officials, primary care physicians, and social services personnel. In addition to oral interviews, written questionnaires may be used.

Before a diagnosis is made, a complete medical checkup may also be recommended to rule out other diseases that could be causing depression-like symptoms. Among the general medical conditions that may cause such symptoms in adolescents are thyroid disease, head injury, anemia, mononucleosis, Lyme disease, chronic fatigue syndrome, hepatitis, and medication side effects. Substance abuse or withdrawal can also cause depression. Of course, when a depressed teenager drinks alcohol or takes drugs, it begs the chicken-and-egg question: Which came first, the substance abuse or the depressed mood? Whatever the answer, however, abused substances may cause or worsen depression by interacting with the brain chemicals that regulate moods.

## How Common Is Adolescent Depression?

It wasn't so long ago that experts were debating whether true depression even existed before adulthood. When a teenager came along whose symptoms were too obvious to ignore, the depression was still often brushed off as ordinary teen moodiness or a trivial problem that the teen would soon outgrow. Since then, we've come a long way toward understanding the nature of adolescent depression. Yes, it does occur, and with surprising frequency. Today, we know that depression often first appears during the adolescent and young adult years. Occasionally, it begins even earlier, striking before puberty. We also know that depression in adolescents can be a long-lasting, recurring, and serious problem, just as it is in adults. However, there is still uncertainty about just how common adolescent depression really is.

To date, some of the most comprehensive data come from the National Comorbidity Survey, which included a nationally representative sample of more than 8,000 Americans between the ages of 15 and 54. In this survey, the researchers found that 14% of young people experienced major depression by the end of adolescence, and another 11% experienced minor depression— a term sometimes used to describe a depressive episode that is similar to major depression but involves fewer symptoms and less impairment in everyday functioning.

A more recent study from the National Institute of Child Health and Human Development found similarly high rates. For this study, researchers gave questionnaires to more than 9,800 students in grades 6, 8, and 10 from schools across the United States. They found that 18% of students reported having some symptoms of depression. The rate of such symptoms was substantially higher in girls (25%) than boys (10%). In both sexes, however, the prevalence of depressive symptoms rose with age. For boys, the prevalence almost doubled between sixth and tenth grades. For girls, it nearly tripled.

**What Role Do Genes Play in Depression?**

Depression doesn't seem to be caused by any single thing. Instead, it appears to result from the complex interplay of genetic, biological, social, and psychological factors combined with stressful life events. As far as genetic influences go, studies have shown that the two most consistent risk factors for major depression are being female and having a family history of the disease.

*Depression doesn't seem to be caused by any single thing.*

In younger children, girls and boys seem to be at about equal risk of having a mood disorder. By adolescence, however, females are two to three times more likely than males to develop depression. In addition, the offspring of depressed parents have a two to four times higher risk of developing the disease themselves than the offspring of nondepressed parents. Children of parents with depression are also more likely to develop depression at an early age and experience recurrent episodes.

Yet, although major depression does seem to run in certain families, it can also occur in individuals with no family history of the disorder. On the flip side, some people whose family tree has depression on nearly every branch manage to go through life without ever developing the disease themselves. At most, then, some parents may pass on a genetic predisposition to depression, which makes their children more vulnerable to environmental risk factors, such as various forms of life stress.

## What Role Does Biology Play in Depression?

Whether depression is genetically based or not, it tends to be associated with changes in brain development, neurochemistry, and function. Unless you happen to be a scientist or doctor, learning about these changes may require getting acquainted with some new terms and concepts. But the effort you invest will be repaid many times over in a greater understanding of your teen's condition. "It's so important for parents to understand about the brain chemicals and parts of the brain that are involved," says one mother, who educated herself and now teaches other parents about the biology of mood disorders.

Modern brain imaging technology allows researchers to take pictures of the living brain at work without the need for surgery. Such studies have found that children and adolescents with depression tend to have significantly smaller-than-average frontal lobes, part of the brain involved in planning, reasoning, controlling voluntary movement, and turning thoughts into words. Specifically, researchers have found less frontal lobe white matter, the inside part of the lobes that is composed largely of the sending branches of nerve cells.

Depression has also been linked to imbalances in certain neurotransmitters, chemicals that act as messengers within the brain. Here's how the process is supposed to work: Nerve cells, called neurons, communicate with each other through a combination of electrical and chemical processes. When a neuron is first activated, it sends an electrical signal from the cell body. This signal travels down a fiberlike branch, called the axon. Once the signal reaches the end of the axon, however, there's a challenge. A tiny gap, called a synapse, exists between each neuron and its neighbors. In order to get the message across this gap, a different delivery method is needed. That's where neurotransmitters come in, since they're able to chemically ferry a message from one neuron to the next.

At this point, then, chemical communication takes over. A neurotransmitter is released from the end of the axon into the synaptic space. There are many different types of neurotransmitters, each with a distinctive chemical shape. A particular kind of neurotransmitter can only be delivered to a matching molecule, called a receptor, on the surface of the receiving neuron. Think of neurotransmitters as keys and receptors as locks. The key has to fit if the message is to be delivered. If it does, the receptor transmits the message into the receiving neuron, where it acts as an on or off switch. If the message is excitatory, it tells the neuron to switch on and continue passing along the signal. If the message is inhibitory, it tells the neuron to switch off and suppress the signal. Either way, a particular message is delivered.

> Think of neurotransmitters as keys and receptors as locks.

Now all that's left is to dispose of the neurotransmitter, which still remains in the synaptic space. One way of doing this is by using enzymes to destroy the neurotransmitter in the synapse. Another is by returning the neurotransmitter to the sending neuron for recycling. A large molecule, called a transporter, carries the neurotransmitter back across the gap to the axon of the neuron that originally sent it. Then the neurotransmitter is absorbed back into the axon that first released it, a process called reuptake. Meanwhile, a complex feedback mechanism tells the sending neuron when to stop sending out more neurotransmitter.

It all adds up to an amazingly efficient process. For people with mood disorders, however, the process seems to go awry. In some cases, the receptors may be either too sensitive or not sensitive enough to a particular neurotransmitter, leading to an excessive or inadequate response. In other cases, the sending cell may release too little of a neurotransmitter, or the transporter molecules may bring it back too soon, before the message has been delivered to the receiving neuron.

Such problems may involve a number of neurotransmitters. Three that have been heavily studied in relation to depression are serotonin, norepinephrine, and dopamine. Serotonin is a neurotransmitter that helps regulate sleep, appetite, and sexual drive. Researchers have found low levels of serotonin in some severely depressed or suicidal individuals, and the most popular antidepressant medications today work by blocking the reuptake of serotonin, thus increasing the brain's supply of this neurotransmitter.

Older types of antidepressant drugs, which are still in use today, increase norepinephrine, either alone or along with serotonin. Norepinephrine plays a role in the body's response to stress, and it helps regulate arousal, sleep, and blood pressure. One older type of antidepressant blocks the reuptake of norepinephrine, while another prevents its breakdown in the synapse. When these drugs were first discovered, scientists reasoned that depression must be caused by low levels of norepinephrine, since the medications are effective for many people. However, they've since learned that the situation is not so cut and dried. It turns out that some people with depression actually have high, rather than low, levels of norepinephrine.

In addition, neither the norepinephrine-boosting drugs nor serotonin antidepressants work for everyone. And even when these types of drug do work, it usually takes several weeks for the full effects to be felt, despite the fact that the drugs begin to have an impact on neurotransmitter levels.

Dopamine is a third neurotransmitter that has been linked to depression. It's essential for movement, and it also influences a person's motivation and perception of reality. Problems with dopamine transmission are associated with the severely distorted thinking seen in psychosis. Dopamine levels also seem to fall during depression and rise during mania in people who cycle back and forth between the two extremes. In addition, depression is a side effect of certain medications (such as the blood pressure drug reserpine) and medical illnesses (such as Parkinson's disease) that reduce the brain's natural dopamine supply.

Just to make matters even more confusing, other brain chemicals have been implicated in depression as well. For example, endorphins are small, protein-like compounds in the brain that have natural pain-relieving and mood-elevating effects similar to those of morphine. Some people with depressive symptoms that fall just short of major depression seem to have low levels of endorphins. Another neurotransmitter called gamma-aminobutyric acid (GABA) inhibits the flow of nerve signals in neurons by blocking the release of other neurotransmitters, such as norepinephrine and dopamine. GABA may also quell anxiety.

Studies have found low levels of GABA in some people with depression.

More research is needed to clarify the specific roles that various neurotransmitters may play in depression. What seems clear already, however, is that depression is a brain disease linked to chemical imbalances, and antidepressant medications help regulate these chemicals. Among other things, researchers are now trying to sort out whether the imbalances are the cause or the effect of depression. Many believe it cuts both ways—in other words, brain chemistry affects behavior, and behavior affects brain chemistry in turn. For example, stress may alter people's brain chemistry, causing them to feel depressed and behave accordingly. However, if these same people alter their behavior by learning to better manage stress, they may be able to further change their brain chemistry in a way that eases depression. It's a fascinating side of the mind-body connection that scientists are just beginning to explore.

*. . . brain chemistry affects behavior, and behavior affects brain chemistry . . .*

## How Does Stress Affect Depression?

Scientifically speaking, stress refers to the body's natural response to any perceived threat—real or imagined, physical or psychological. The threat initially sets off alarm bells inside the brain. In response, the brain orders the release of certain hormones that prepare the body to fight or flee. As the body goes into a state of high alert, a person's heart rate, blood pressure, breathing rate, metabolism, and muscle tension all increase. This rapid response system can be a lifesaver in a true emergency, because it allows the person to react quickly and effectively. However, when stress is frequent or prolonged, the physiological wear and tear can take a toll on mind and body alike. One possible consequence is depression. In children and adolescents, as in adults, research has found a strong link between depression and stressful life events.

Stress is in the mind of the beholder, however. The experience of stress depends on an individual's appraisal of a situation as threatening, and different people may differ in how they size up the same situation. It's not surprising, then, that no one type of event invariably leads to depression. Many young people bounce back from terrible loss or adversity with surprising resilience. On the other hand, when depression does occur, it isn't always traceable to a single big trauma. Instead, it often seems to be related to the cumulative impact of many smaller events.

That being said, certain life events in adolescence do indeed raise the risk of depression, although individual teenagers may be more or less susceptible to their effects. One particularly powerful source of stress for teens is the loss of a parent through death or permanent separation. Other common sources of teen stress include physical or emotional abuse, sexual assault, bullying, poverty, or a personal disappointment, such as a romantic breakup.

Stress and genes may also converge in families where more than one member has a mood disorder. For example, one mother of a 14-year-old son with bipolar disorder says her 11-year-old daughter was recently diagnosed with depression, and she believes that her daughter's symptoms were partly triggered by the stress of dealing with their chaotic family life. "That's what happens when you have more than one child who's predisposed to a mood disorder," she says. "One child goes off, and it sets everybody else in motion."

## Does Early Life Stress Have a Lasting Effect?

The past can influence the present, too. A large body of research now suggests that stress experienced early in life can continue to exert an effect lasting all the way into adulthood. To understand how this may work, it helps to know a bit more about how stress affects the brain and body. When a person is faced with a threat, it activates the hypothalamus, part of the brain that serves as the command center for the nervous and hormonal systems. The hypothalamus releases a substance called corticotropin-releasing factor (CRF). The CRF travels to the pituitary gland, located at the base of the brain, where it triggers the release of adrenocorticotropic hormone (ACTH). Then ACTH travels to the adrenal glands, located just above the kidneys, where it stimulates the release of a powerful hormone called cortisol. This hormone, in turn, is responsible for many of the physiological effects of stress.

> . . . stress experienced early in life can continue to exert an effect lasting all the way into adulthood.

Taken together, these elements make up a body system known as the hypothalamic-pituitary-adrenal (HPA) axis. This system seems to play an important role in depression. Since the late 1960s, hundreds of studies have shown that people with depression who are not on medication, especially those with the most severe symptoms, tend to show increased activity in the HPA axis. Specifically, the brain cells that produce CRF seem to be overactive, which may explain other changes seen in depressed people, such as enlargement of the pituitary and adrenal glands and high levels of cortisol in the urine, blood, and spinal fluid.

According to one theory, extreme stress early in childhood, when brain pathways are still developing, may affect the CRF-producing brain cells in a way that leads to long-lasting overactivity. This, in turn, may lead to a super-sensitive stress response, in which the brain cells react vigorously to even mild threats.

Ultimately, the price paid for this overactive stress response may be depression.

It's worth noting, however, that most of the evidence to date supporting this theory comes from studies in animals or in human adults. The findings in human adolescents have been less dramatic. For example, brain scans have shown that part of the brain called the hippocampus—an area that plays a role in learning, memory, and emotion—actually tends to be smaller in grown women who have depression than in those who aren't depressed. The same size difference isn't seen in abused children or adolescents, though, leading some researchers to suggest that it's the repeated bursts of cortisol over a long period of time that may eventually cause the hippocampus to shrink.

CRF is also found in parts of the brain outside the HPA axis. The brain pathways that carry CRF elsewhere in the brain link with neurons that release serotonin and norepinephrine—two neurotransmitters involved in depression. Scientists are still trying to figure out exactly how all the pieces of the puzzle fit together. However, the picture that is emerging reveals that depression is not just in someone's mind. It's also in the person's brain, where it is associated with very real physical abnormalities.

## What Social Factors Are Related to Depression?

One of the biggest fears many parents harbor is that they somehow caused their child's depression by providing a less-than-perfect home environment. As one mother put it, "You start second-guessing yourself, asking, 'Should I have done something differently? Did I pay her enough attention? Did I give in too fast when she had temper tantrums?'" The fact is, 100% of teenagers would probably be depressed if parental perfection were the only way to prevent it.

"You start second-guessing yourself . . ."

That's not to say that a warm, stable home isn't a powerfully positive force in any young person's life. But depression is a complex disease with multiple causes, and parenting is only one of many factors that may affect it. Children raised by loving, attentive, competent parents can become depressed, just as they can develop other diseases.

However, it's also true that one of the main problems prompting parents to seek help for their depressed teenagers is an increase in family arguments and conflict. In some cases, this may reflect a preexisting pattern of troubled relationships. Beginning as far back as infancy, an inconsistent or inattentive parenting style may make it harder for children to learn how to form healthy, secure emotional attachments. This, in turn, may lead to an insecure, self-critical view of themselves and the world that provides fertile ground for later depression. As children get older, they are also more likely to become depressed if their parents are very critical, rejecting, or controlling. Not surprisingly, traumatic events—such as the death of or separation from a parent; mental illness in a parent; severe neglect; or physical, emotional, or sexual abuse—just increase the risk further.

Yet family dysfunction is a two-way street. Living with a teenager can be challenging under the best of circumstances. When the teen is exceptionally irritable, gloomy, or apathetic as a result of depression, the difficulties increase exponentially. It's easy to become trapped in a vicious cycle, in which the teen's depression-related behavior creates conflict within the family, which increases the depression, which causes more conflict, and so on. Fortunately, treatment for the teen's depression, perhaps combined with family therapy, can help break the cycle.

Of course, family members aren't the only influences on a teenager's life. At this age, friends are extremely important as well. As a general rule, however, depressed teens tend to have trouble making and keeping friends. Many wind up feeling like outcasts at school, which just adds to their emotional burden. Others end up as either the victims of bullies or bullies themselves. One large study found that young people who were involved in bullying, whether as victims or as perpetrators, were twice as likely to report having depressive symptoms as those who weren't involved. Once again, appropriate treatment for depression, possibly including social skills training, can help a teenager learn to relate more positively to others.

## What Psychological Factors Are Related to Depression?

Scientifically speaking, temperament refers to a person's inborn tendency to react to events in a particular way. In essence, this boils down to personality traits that first become apparent in infancy or early childhood and that tend to last throughout the life span. Such traits help dictate how a person responds to any given situation. Some studies have found that young people who are generally shy, withdrawn, or easily upset may have an increased risk of depression.

Another line of thinking holds that people who have a generally pessimistic view of themselves, the world, and their future are more likely to become depressed. Known as the cognitive theory of depression, this theory is based on the observation that some people habitually view the world as a threatening place and themselves as powerless to cope with many situations. Such people tend to blame themselves for negative events, even ones beyond their control. They also tend to believe that the negative circumstances will last a long time and undercut whatever they do.

It's easy to see how this kind of pessimistic thinking style could increase the stress that people feel in all kinds of situations. This, in turn, might trigger or worsen depression in vulnerable individuals. Indeed, a number of studies now support this theory. Interestingly, studies have also found that the likelihood of a negative thinking style increases as young people move from early childhood to late childhood to adolescence. It's probably no coincidence that this parallels the increasing risk of depression during those same years. One popular form of psychotherapy, called cognitive-behavioral therapy, is geared toward helping people learn to identify and replace the unreasonably negative beliefs that may contribute to their depression.

## What Other Conditions Often Coexist With Depression?

As we've seen, depression is a multifaceted problem that touches virtually every aspect of a person's life. It should come as no surprise, then, that most adolescents with depression have other emotional, behavioral, and learning problems as well. These coexisting disorders—known as comorbid conditions in psychiatric lingo—may confuse the picture and make treatment more complicated.

*. . . most adolescents with depression have other emotional, behavioral, and learning problems as well.*

Nevertheless, it's very important that they be recognized and addressed in their own right. Below are some of the conditions that often occur side by side with depression in adolescents.

- Anxiety disorders—More than 60% of depressed adolescents have had an anxiety disorder, either in the past or at the same time as their depression. In one common pattern, an anxiety disorder starts before puberty, followed by major depression in adolescence. While it's perfectly normal for young people to feel a little worried or nervous at times, those with anxiety disorders experience overwhelming anxiety or fear that interferes with their ability to function in daily life. Anxiety disorders come in several different forms, but they all involve extreme or maladaptive feelings of tension, fear, or worry.

- Substance abuse—Abuse of alcohol or other drugs is common in adolescents with depression. While substance abuse itself can cause depressive symptoms, there are other times when the depression comes first, and teens turn to drinking or drug use in an effort to escape their mental pain. Unfortunately, substance abuse just makes the situation worse, so it's imperative that teens be treated for both conditions. Cigarette smoking is often associated with depression as well.

- Eating disorders—From one-third to one-half of all people with eating disorders also suffer from depression. Most of these individuals are adolescent girls or young women, and some studies suggest that there may be a stronger association with dysthymia than with major depression. People with eating disorders may severely restrict what they eat, or they may go on eating binges, then attempt to compensate by such means as self-induced vomiting or misuse of laxatives.

- Attention-deficit hyperactivity disorder (ADHD)—It's not uncommon for adolescents with depression to also have ADHD. The primary characteristics of ADHD are inattention, hyperactivity, or impulsive behavior that begins early in life and may continue throughout the school years. Some children are bothered mainly by distractibility and a short attention span, others by hyperactivity and impulsiveness, and still others by all these problems combined. The symptoms may resolve by late adolescence, but they often last into adulthood.

- Conduct disorder—Most teenagers test the rules now and then. However, those with conduct disorder have extreme difficulty following the rules or conforming to social norms. They may threaten others, get into fights, set fires, vandalize property, lie, steal, stay out all night, or run away from home. In adolescents, depression and conduct disorder often go hand in hand. Such teenagers frequently are labeled "bad" or delinquent rather than mentally ill, and some may wind up being written off as lost causes rather than getting the help they need.

- Oppositional defiant disorder—Most adolescents also defy authority at times, especially when they're tired, stressed, or upset. However, for those with oppositional defiant disorder, the defiant, uncooperative, and hostile behavior becomes a long-lasting way of life. Symptoms may include angry outbursts, excessive arguing with adults, habitual refusal to comply with adult requests, and deliberate attempts to annoy people. It's tempting to hope that a teen acting this way is just "going through a stage" and will soon grow out of it. However, extremely oppositional behavior is a serious problem that shouldn't be ignored. Studies suggest that from one-third to one-half of all adolescents who die by suicide have either oppositional defiant disorder or conduct disorder, often in conjunction with depression.

> It's tempting to hope that a teen acting this way is just "going through a stage"

- Learning disorders—Some young people with depression have a learning disorder, too. Such disorders affect their performance in school or their ability to function in everyday situations that require reading, writing, or math skills. Depression itself can make it very difficult for students to pay attention in class, and it can sap them of the energy and motivation they need to study and do homework. As a result, grades may plummet, and school attendance may falter. When a learning disorder is added to the mix, the situation becomes even more challenging. Both treatment for the depression and academic intervention for the learning problem may be needed to get the student back on track at school.

As a practical matter, it can sometimes be very hard to tell whether a particular teen's behavior is due to depression, another disorder, or garden-variety rebellion. "My daughter's skipping classes like crazy in high school," one father says. "Is that some consequence of the depression? Some failure to adjust, some lack of maturity related to the illness?" Perhaps. Or the same behavior might be caused by substance abuse, conduct disorder, or oppositional defiant disorder. Or it might be due to a condition—such as social anxiety, hyperactivity, or a learning disorder—that makes going to class an agony. An experienced mental health professional can help sort out the problems, which is the first step to finding solutions.

Additional information about these various conditions may be obtained from the sources listed in the Resources for Related Problems section (pp. 186–187) of this book.

### What Is the Outlook for the Future?

"Just because you have this disorder doesn't mean you can't be extremely productive," says Carol. She should know: Carol, her husband, and both of their children have depression or bipolar disorder. "You just have to stay on top of things," she adds. "Yeah, we obviously have our ups and downs—no pun intended. But if we have a setback, we brush ourselves off and get right back on the horse."

Each individual's experience of depression is unique. The course of a particular adolescent's illness depends on many factors, such as how severe the symptoms are and whether he or she gets appropriate treatment. It's safe to say, however, that the depression isn't going to disappear overnight. This is a serious disease, and recovery can take some time. Left to run its course without treatment, an episode of major depression lasts about 7 to 9 months, on average. After one year, naturalistic studies suggest that 40% of affected people will still have major depression, and an additional 20% will have some depressive symptoms.

Then there is the problem of recurrence after the first bout of depression has finally come to an end. About 60% of people who have a single episode of depression go on to have another. After two episodes, the odds of a third are even higher, and after three episodes, the chances of a fourth rise to 90%. In the course of a lifetime, people who don't get treatment average five to seven episodes of major depression, and the episodes tend to get worse each time.

Fortunately, treatments such as medication, psychotherapy, or a combination of both can improve the outlook considerably. If treatment is started early, it may help keep depression from ever becoming chronic or severe. Treatment can also interrupt the downward spiral into frequent recurrences. In addition, it can alleviate symptoms and potentially prevent the most-dreaded consequence of all: suicide.

If you think your adolescent may be suffering from depression, it's wise to seek professional help promptly, even if your teen doesn't want it or insists that nothing is wrong. You know what's normal and what's not for your child, so trust your instincts. At the very least, you may prevent needless mental pain and suffering. At most, you might save your teen's life.

. . . trust your instincts.

## A Dose of Hope

What does the future hold? Will your child ever be able to go to college or get a good job? No one can predict the future with certainty, of course, but there are plenty of very good reasons to be hopeful. Here are three: Television journalist Jane Pauley, psychiatry professor Kay Redfield Jamison, and Pulitzer Prize-winning novelist William Styron are among the well-known individuals who have risen to the top of their professions despite struggling with depression or bipolar disorder. They've shared their stories in these memoirs, which are sometimes disturbing, but ultimately quite encouraging.

Jamison, Kay Redfield. *An Unquiet Mind: A Memoir of Moods and Madness.* New York: Alfred A. Knopf, 1995.

Pauley, Jane. *Skywriting: A Life Out of the Blue.* New York: Random House, 2004.

Styron, William. *Darkness Visible: A Memoir of Madness.* New York: Random House, 1990.

## Bipolar Disorder: Characteristics, Causes, and Risk Factors; Other Conditions; Outlook for the Future

When you look back on being a teenager, you may have fond memories of the physical energy and emotional intensity you possessed then—and perhaps wish you could recapture now. For teens with bipolar disorder, however, that energy is cranked up to an excessively, sometimes excruciatingly, high level. This overly high, manic state is the defining characteristic of bipolar disorder. In some cases, the mania alternates with bouts of depression. In other cases, the disease starts with mania alone, or the mania and depression are mixed together at the same time. Many teens experience milder mood swings, but those with bipolar disorder are whipsawed between extremes. The highs are much too high, and the falls can be brutal.

If you're the parent of an adolescent with bipolar disorder, you don't have to be told how exhausting it is to try to keep up with someone whose thoughts and behavior are racing at high speed. The difficulty of your situation is only compounded by the well-meaning but ill-informed attitudes you're apt to encounter, even among some professionals who ought to know better. You may hear that the only true bipolar disorder is the type that conforms to the classic pattern of distinct highs alternating with distinct lows. Or you may be assured that bipolar disorder never occurs before late adolescence, and there's nothing wrong with your child that a firm hand won't cure. In your heart, you may know this isn't so, but it's still hard to encounter skepticism and disapproval when what you really need is information and support. There are several reasons why bipolar disorder in adolescents is so widely misunderstood. One is that it occurs less often than depression. Another is the fact that doctors and researchers have only recently realized that bipolar disorder can look quite different in children and young adolescents than it does in older adolescents and adults. Rather than distinct up and down phases, youngsters often have an ongoing mood disturbance that is a mix of mania and depression. The rapid cycling between moods can lead to great irritability, and the continuous nature of the mood disturbance may mean that there are few well periods between episodes.

A third source of confusion is the surface similarity between the childhood form of bipolar disorder and ADHD. Since ADHD is more common, it's only logical that doctors would suspect it first when confronted with a young person who is distractible, restless, and impulsive. It can take considerable professional experience to tell the two conditions apart. In addition, some doctors may lean toward a diagnosis of ADHD in a misguided effort to shield a youngster from the stigma of mental illness. The problem with this approach is that it also keeps the child from getting appropriate treatment.

It is only since the 1990s that child and adolescent psychiatrists have begun diagnosing bipolar disorder with greater frequency in their young patients. Before that, there was strong resistance within the medical and mental health community to the idea that bipolar disorder even existed before the late teen years. Many nonspecialist professionals, including some psychiatrists who treat mainly adults, may still have catching up to do with the latest thinking. Getting an accurate diagnosis for an adolescent with bipolar disorder may require seeking out the most knowledgeable, up-to-date professionals—all the more reason that parents need to be actively involved in finding the best care for their teens.

## What Is Mania?

Bipolar disorder is actually a spectrum of symptoms that vary in the intensity of the highs as well as the presence, intensity, and timing of the lows. The one thing that all bipolar conditions have in common, however, is some degree of mania. Essentially, this is an overly high or irritable mood that lasts for at least a week or leads to dangerous behavior. It causes symptoms such as an exaggerated sense of self-importance, decreased need for sleep, increased talkativeness or activity, or risk-taking behavior. In young people, mania sometimes also takes the form of extreme irritability or explosive tantrums.

## What Is Hypomania?

At times, people with bipolar disorder experience a more moderate level of mania, called hypomania. Those who are in a hypomanic state may feel unusually good or cheerful, and some

# Mania

Below are the *DSM-IV-TR* criteria for a manic episode:

1. An overly high, expansive, or irritable mood must be present for at least 1 week. The time period can be shorter if the symptoms are severe enough to require hospitalization.

2. At least three of the following symptoms must occur during the same period. If the person's mood is only irritable, rather than high or expansive, a minimum of four symptoms must be present.

   a. Inflated self-esteem or grandiose ideas about oneself (for example, feeling all-important or like a superhero with special powers)

   b. Decreased need for sleep

   c. Talkativeness or a feeling of pressure to keep talking

   d. Abrupt changes of topic during speech or racing thoughts

   e. Being easily distractible

   f. Increased activity

   g. Excessive involvement in pleasurable but high-risk activities (for example, driving recklessly, having promiscuous sex, or going on spending sprees)

3. The mood disturbance causes marked impairment in functioning or relationships, or it is severe enough to necessitate hospitalization or lead to psychotic symptoms, such as delusional thinking or hallucinations.

4. The symptoms are not due to the direct physiological effects of alcohol or drug abuse, a general medical condition, or the side effects of a medication.

Adapted from American Psychiatric Association, *Diagnostic and Statistical Manual of Mental Disorders* (4th ed., text revision, p. 362). Washington, DC: American Psychiatric Association, 2000.

---

# Hypomania

Below are the *DSM-IV-TR* criteria for a hypomanic episode:

1. A somewhat high, expansive, or irritable mood must be present for at least 4 days. The mood should be clearly different from the person's usual mood when not depressed.

2. At least three of the symptoms of mania must occur during the same period. If the person's mood is only irritable, rather than high or expansive, four symptoms of mania should be present.

3. The change in mood should be noticeable to others. However, it is not severe enough to cause marked impairment, necessitate hospitalization, or lead to psychotic symptoms.

4. The symptoms are not due to the direct physiological effects of alcohol or drug abuse, a general medical condition, or the side effects of a medication.

---

Adapted from American Psychiatric Association, *Diagnostic and Statistical Manual of Mental Disorders* (4th ed., text revision, p. 368). Washington, DC: American Psychiatric Association, 2000.

---

may be exceptionally productive or creative. As a result, even after family and friends learn to recognize the warning signs of hypomania, the person who is going through it may insist that nothing is wrong. Without treatment, however, hypomania can escalate into full-blown mania or switch into depression.

## What Is a Mixed Episode?

Other people with bipolar disorder may experience mixed episodes. This type of episode is exactly what it sounds like: a mixture of mania and depression occurring at the same time, rather than one after the other. For some with bipolar disorder, a mixed episode is merely a transitional state as mania switches to depression. For others, however, a mix of symptoms is the primary way that bipolar illness manifests itself. The latter pattern is particularly common in children and young adolescents.

## Mixed Episode

Below are the *DSM-IV-TR* criteria for a mixed episode:

1. The criteria for both mania and major depression are met nearly every day for at least 1 week. Although young people often experience a mix of simultaneous symptoms, many fail to meet the criteria for full-blown depression, so their condition is not technically considered a mixed episode.

2. The mood disturbance causes marked impairment in functioning or relationships, or it is severe enough to necessitate hospitalization or lead to psychotic symptoms, such as delusional thinking or hallucinations.

3. The symptoms are not due to the direct physiological effects of alcohol or drug abuse, a general medical condition, or the side effects of a medication.

Adapted from American Psychiatric Association, *Diagnostic and Statistical Manual of Mental Disorders* (4th ed., text revision, p. 365). Washington, DC: American Psychiatric Association, 2000.

## What Are the Different Bipolar Illnesses?

The mood episodes of bipolar disorder can fall into a variety of patterns:

- Bipolar I—This disorder is characterized by the occurrence of at least one manic or mixed episode. Often, but not always, it has been preceded by an episode of major depression. About 10% to 15% of adolescents who have had recurrent bouts of major depression go on to develop bipolar I. After a first brush with mania, more than 90% of people have more episodes in the future.

- Bipolar II—The essential feature of this disorder is an alternating pattern of hypomania and major depression. For people who have struggled with deep depression for some time, the ordinary good feelings that arise once the depression finally lifts may feel a little strange at first. Such individuals may just need some time to readjust to feeling happy again. This isn't necessarily cause for alarm unless the new mood rises to the level of hypomania. After a first bout of full-blown mania, the diagnosis automatically changes to bipolar I.

- Cyclothymia—This is a long-lasting mood disorder that causes cycling between hypomania and relatively mild depressive symptoms. For a diagnosis of adolescent cyclothymia to be made, the pattern must have lasted for at least a year. Although there may be intermittent periods of normal mood, they never last for more than 2 months at a time during the illness. There is a 15% to 50% risk that a person with cyclothymia will later develop bipolar I or bipolar II.

- Bipolar not otherwise specified—This catchall category includes several possibilities. For example, there might be alternating mood episodes that fulfill all the requirements for mania or major depression except the ones pertaining to duration. Or there might be recurrent episodes of hypomania without alternating periods of depression. BP-NOS, as it's often abbreviated, may actually be the most common bipolar diagnosis in children and young adolescents. That's because the *DSM-IV-TR* criteria are based mainly on adults, and young people may show a slightly different pattern of symptoms. For instance, they often develop a mixture of mania and depression that doesn't quite qualify as a mixed episode.

*BP-NOS . . . may actually be the most common bipolar diagnosis*

## Can Bipolar Disorder Take Different Forms?

The various bipolar illnesses can be further divided into different subtypes. A severe episode of mania, like a severe bout of major depression, can be considered psychotic if it produces delusions or hallucinations. For example, manic teens might have delusions that they possess superhuman powers or hear voices telling them how remarkably superior they are. An episode of mania can be said to have catatonic features if it includes symptoms such as physical immobility, stupor, purposeless overactivity, extreme negativism, peculiar mannerisms, or parrot-like repetition of someone else's words.

In addition, bipolar I or bipolar II can be designated as rapid cycling if four or more mood episodes occur within a single year. These episodes are separated either by periods of relative wellness or by a distinct switch from high to low moods. In adults, rapid cycling is the exception rather than the rule, occurring in about 10% to 20% of people with bipolar disorder. In children and young adolescents, though, the reverse appears to be true. When bipolar disorder begins at such an early age, it usually seems to be rapid cycling and continuous.

In some cases, the moods cycle every few days or even several times within a single day. It's easy to see how this could lead to a jumble of moods, with symptoms of both mania and depression occurring at once. On the manic side, the result is often irritability, restlessness, agitation, rage, tantrums, and even violence rather than the euphoria or elation seen in adults.

### What Warning Signs Should You Watch For?

Bipolar disorder can include both manic and depressive symptoms. While both types of symptoms may be quite serious, the manic ones are apt to be more attention grabbing. It's not uncommon for young people in the grips of mania to experience bouts of explosive rage, often directed against family members. Some throw tantrums that last for hours, others wreck their rooms, and still others threaten their parents or siblings. You're not likely to miss this sort of irritable mania, but it can be difficult to differentiate from other, more common emotional and behavioral disorders.

*It's not uncommon for young people in the grips of mania to experience bouts of explosive rage . . .*

"She started acting up, causing trouble at day camp," one mother says of her daughter with bipolar disorder, who was 13 years old at the time. "She was being defiant, doing weird things, lashing out. When they called me, she didn't want to be picked up, so she ran off screaming and yelling. She climbed on top of this tall structure and was banging her head on it to beat the craziness out of her head—those were her words." It's easy to see how this kind of behavior can be confusing and frightening for all concerned, including the teen herself.

On the other hand, some adolescents may develop a manic state that closely resembles the mania seen in adults. Rather than irritable, they may feel unnaturally elated, full of ideas, and super-energized. While this might not sound so bad, it can quickly escalate to the point where the teens feel overwhelmed by their uncontrollable thoughts and impulses. Under the influence of mania, they may also make some extremely risky or self-destructive choices.

However it manifests itself, bipolar disorder doesn't develop overnight. Instead, research suggests that it may be a progressive illness that grows gradually worse over time. Early on, the symptoms may be milder and less protracted than they are farther down the line. The symptoms also tend to be easier to treat effectively before the disease is well established. If you think your teen may be at risk, it's wise to seek help sooner rather than later. Be alert for these warning signs:

• Behavior that is extremely irritable, or overly silly and elated

- Unrealistically high opinion of oneself or one's abilities
- Challenging adult authority
- Great increase in energy
- Being able to go for days with little or no sleep without feeling tired
- Speech that is too much, too fast, changes topic too quickly, or cannot be interrupted
- Attention that darts constantly from one thing to the next
- Repeated high-risk behavior, such as substance abuse, reckless driving, or sexual promiscuity
- Increased sexual thoughts, feelings, or behavior
- Any of the warning signs of depression

---

### A Parent's-Eye View of Mania

Here's how five parents describe mania in their adolescent children:

"My son was hit by a car once, just wandering in the road at night. It was a young girl that hit him, and I guess it scared the heck out of her. But he was fine, and he thought it was the coolest thing ever."

"One Sunday, she started smashing every glass object in her room. Then she went and squirted toothpaste all over the bathroom."

"I've been in Wal-Mart when my daughter went off and lost it. The entire store kind of came to a halt as they watched this screaming kid."

"The stereo's on, the TV's on, the computer's on, he's talking on the phone. He could do everything all at once and know what was going on everywhere—*and* hear voices in the basement, or so he told me."

"Instead of terrible twos, we've got terrible fifteens."

---

### How Is Bipolar Disorder Diagnosed?

The diagnosis of bipolar disorder in an adolescent is no easy matter. As already noted, young people may not display the classic pattern of symptoms seen in adults, and the symptoms they do have often look similar to those of more common emotional and behavioral problems. If bipolar disorder is present but goes undiagnosed, the young person may suffer needlessly, now and in the future. If it's misdiagnosed as something else, the adolescent may be prescribed a medication that actually makes the mania worse. And if bipolar disorder is diagnosed when it isn't really present, the adolescent may be treated with medications that are ineffective for the real problem. Finding a doctor who can make a correct diagnosis is crucial.

*Finding a doctor who can make a correct diagnosis is crucial.*

Both bipolar disorder and ADHD can lead to inattentiveness, hyperactivity, and impulsiveness. Unfortunately, there is no handy lab test or brain scan to differentiate the two. Instead, mental health professionals must become psychiatric detectives. These are some of the clues they look for:

- Angry outbursts—Like anyone else, adolescents with ADHD may get angry, but they generally calm down within half an hour. In those with bipolar disorder, however, the anger may last for up to 4 hours.
- Destructiveness—Adolescents with ADHD may break things, but it's usually an accident caused by inattentiveness. In contrast, those with bipolar disorder may destroy property intentionally in a fit of rage.

Since psychotic symptoms are relatively common in adolescent bipolar disorder, the condition is also sometimes confused with other psychotic illnesses, especially schizophrenia or schizoaffective disorder. Any of these conditions can produce delusional beliefs that are wildly out of touch with reality or hallucinations such as hearing voices that aren't really there. In addition, both bipolar disorder and schizoaffective disorder involve major mood swings. One key difference is that, in bipolar disorder, psychotic symptoms tend to occur during the worst periods of mood disturbance. In schizoaffective disorder, on the other hand, psychotic symptoms remain even when the moods settle down. Since the disorders differ in treatment and outcome, an accurate diagnosis is important.

As with depression, the presence or absence of symptoms is assessed through interviews with the adolescent, parents, and other adults who may be familiar with the young person's lifestyle and behavior. In addition to oral interviews, written questionnaires may be used. When meeting with your child's doctor for the first time, come prepared to describe the nature, severity, duration, and timing of the symptoms you've observed in as much detail as possible. Since bipolar disorder seems to have a strong genetic component, you will probably also be asked about family members with mental illness or bipolar-type mood swings.

Before a diagnosis is made, a complete medical checkup may also be in order. The goal is to rule out general medical conditions that can mimic mania or depression, such as certain hormonal disorders, neurological conditions, and infectious diseases. Medication side effects are also considered. Among other possibilities, the stimulants used to treat ADHD and the antidepressants used to treat depression can sometimes trigger a manic episode. In addition, several commonly abused drugs can also produce symptoms of mania, including anabolic steroids, amphetamines, cocaine, phenycyclidine (PCP), inhalants, and MDMA (ecstasy).

**How Common Is Adolescent Bipolar Disorder?**

Given the challenges involved in diagnosing bipolar disorder, it's not surprising that precise data on its frequency during adolescence are lacking. Studies have found that about 1% of American adults have bipolar I. Unlike depression, this disorder seems to be about equally common in males and females. In addition, it seems that about 1% to 3% of adults may suffer from other types of bipolar illnesses. The rate in older teenagers seems to be similar. The best available data suggest that 1.0% to 1.3% of 15- to 18-year-olds have experienced at least one episode of mania. In addition, one study sponsored by the National Institutes of Health found that close to 6% of adolescents may have some manic symptoms that don't rise to the level of mania or hypomania.

One thing that does seem clear from the research is that adult bipolar disorder frequently has its roots in adolescence or even before. In some surveys, 20% to 40% of adults with bipolar disorder say that their illness began in childhood. Often, the first manifestation is major depression, dysthymia, or cyclothymia. Anxiety and disruptive behaviors may also occur at this early stage. If things are allowed to run their course, however, bipolar I or bipolar II may eventually develop.

## What Role Do Genes Play in Bipolar Disorder?

The most consistent risk factor for bipolar disorder is family history. Studies have shown that the chance of eventually developing bipolar disorder is about 15% to 30% for individuals who have a sibling or one parent with the disease. The odds rise to 50% to 75% for those who have two bipolar parents, and 70% for those with a bipolar identical twin. While genes are clearly important, however, they aren't the whole explanation. If they were, the identical twin of someone with the illness would *always* develop it, too. As it actually happens, however, some identical twins and others whose genetic risk seems quite high never develop bipolar disorder.

Research to date suggests that bipolar disorder probably involves multiple genes. As with other illnesses, having a particular genetic variant doesn't automatically mean you'll develop the condition. For one thing, the gene may be modified by other variations in the person's genetic makeup. In addition, the fact that the onset of bipolar disorder is so unpredictable indicates that environmental factors also play a major role in this disease. At present, there is still much to be learned about the way various genes and the environment interact to cause bipolar disorder.

One interesting side note is that, in each generation since World War II, the age of onset for bipolar disorder has apparently grown younger. The reason for these changes is still unknown. To some extent, they may simply reflect heightened awareness of the disease. However, the changes might also be due in part to an inheritance pattern within families called anticipation. In this pattern, there is a tendency for individuals in successive generations to develop genetic disorders at earlier ages and with more severe symptoms. Anticipation is often seen in disorders caused by a certain type of genetic mutation that tends to increase in size and have a more significant effect with each passing generation. Whether anticipation is actually present in bipolar disorder remains a matter of some debate, however.

*"I have 10 family members who take medication for various mood disorders . . . my son is just one of us."*

The genetic component of bipolar disorder means that many adolescents with the disorder may have relatives who share the illness. There can be a definite upside to this situation if the relatives serve as positive role models. Lisa, a mother who is diagnosed with bipolar disorder and has a teenage son with the same diagnosis, explains how it works in her family: "I refer to it as Wilson Personality Disorder. I have 10 family members who take medications for various mood disorders, so we call ourselves the chemically enhanced Wilsons—there's nothing negative about it. And my son is just one of us. I think that does help him, because he's never felt ostracized."

## What Role Does Biology Play in Bipolar Disorder?

Few studies have been done comparing the brain structure of adolescents with and without bipolar disorder. In adults, however, studies using sophisticated imaging techniques have found that the brains of people with bipolar disorder tend to differ from the brains of healthy individuals. Among the differences that have been found are:

- Small, abnormal areas in white matter, a form of matter inside the brain that is composed largely of the sending branches of nerve cells
- Decreased number of nerve cells in part of the hippocampus, a structure in the brain that plays a role in learning, memory, and emotion
- Decreased number and density of support cells in the prefrontal cortex, part of the brain involved in complex thought, problem solving, and emotion

The different phases of bipolar disorder also appear to be associated with imbalances in the chemicals that brain cells use to communicate. A number of biochemical changes linked to major depression are discussed in the Depression section (pp. 18–22) of this chapter. Studies have also noted reduced activity in the prefrontal cortex during the depressive phase of bipolar disorder. Meanwhile, other biochemical changes, which are less well understood, may be related to mania. Lithium, a medication that is widely used for treating bipolar disorder, is thought to work by bringing the various brain chemicals into better balance.

What is the exact significance of these findings? Researchers are still trying to sort that out. It may be many years before the physiology and biochemistry underlying bipolar disorder are truly understood. However, enough is already known to make it clear that bipolar disorder is a very real disease originating in the brain, the same way that Alzheimer's disease and Parkinson's disease are.

### How Does Stress Affect Bipolar Disorder?

As far back as 1921, Emil Kraepelin, the German psychiatrist who first defined bipolar disorder as we know it today, noted that initial episodes of mania or depression were often brought on by stressful life events. As time went on, however, less and less stress was needed to trigger an episode. Eventually, episodes might begin to occur spontaneously, with no apparent trigger at all.

One modern theory advanced to explain this effect is known as the kindling hypothesis. It states that the first episode of mania or depression may spark long-lasting changes in the brain that make it more sensitive to future stress. Kindling helps explain why mood disorders tend to get worse over time, and why less and less seems to be needed to set off an episode. This raises the possibility that early treatment for mood symptoms might prevent the increased sensitivity that leads to later attacks. More research is needed to confirm whether this actually occurs. However, it seems quite plausible that prompt treatment of adolescent bipolar disorder might not only reduce suffering now but also change the course of the illness in the future.

## What Social Factors Are Related to Bipolar Disorder?

Bipolar disorder is based inside a person's brain, but outside events may set it in motion. Adolescents with bipolar disorder frequently have trouble getting along with their parents and siblings. The teens' own erratic behavior may, in turn, intensify any conflict that already exists within the family. This can set up a cycle of escalating stress and tension that may be a trigger for symptoms.

Research also suggests that disruptions in daily routine may trigger mania in some individuals. People with bipolar disorder seem to have very delicate internal clocks. When something happens to throw off their daily rhythms, the result may be an episode of mania. Sleep deprivation seems to be the culprit many cases. As the mother of a 17-year-old daughter with bipolar disorder explains, "She would stay up all night, then try to function during the day, which aggravated her symptoms." For this reason, many doctors recommend that their patients with bipolar disorder stick to a structured daily routine and sleep schedule. When this approach is combined with medication, it may help people keep their moods in better balance.

*"She would stay up all night, then try to function during the day, which aggravated her symptoms."*

## What Other Conditions Often Coexist With Bipolar Disorder?

Bipolar disorder doesn't exist in a vacuum. Instead, it often exists side by side with other emotional and behavioral disorders. These comorbid conditions, as they're called, make diagnosis and treatment more complicated. Since they may play a

*Bipolar disorder doesn't exist in a vacuum . . .*

big role in causing or maintaining a particular adolescent's problems, though, it's crucial that they be recognized and treated. Following are some of the conditions that often occur alongside bipolar disorder in adolescents.

- ADHD—Studies have found that 60% to 90% of individuals with childhood mania may have ADHD as well. Young people with both bipolar disorder and ADHD are prone to hyperactivity, distractibility, impulsiveness, decreased need for sleep, irritability, and temper tantrums. Given the many similarities, the potential for misdiagnosis is high. In fact, the overlap is so great that some experts question whether childhood mania and ADHD are really separate entities at all. However, most agree that there are subtle but significant distinctions between the two. For example, dangerous behavior by an adolescent with bipolar disorder often seems to be intentional, while the same behavior by a teen with ADHD is more typically caused by inattentiveness. A complex blend of the two behavior patterns may be seen in adolescents who have both bipolar disorder and ADHD at once.

- Conduct disorder—This disorder is characterized by extreme difficulty following the rules or behaving in a socially acceptable way. Conduct disorder is strongly associated with bipolar disorder in young people. In fact, studies have found that up to two-thirds of young people with mania may have conduct disorder as well. As with ADHD, the similarities between the two conditions are so great that it can be hard to tell them apart. One differentiating factor is the presence of guilt. Youngsters with bipolar disorder often feel guilty, even when there's no reason to feel this way. In contrast, those with conduct disorder usually feel no remorse, even when they've done something wrong. By the same token, adolescents with bipolar disorder may be irrationally paranoid, while those with conduct disorder frequently have very good reason to believe that someone is out to get even with them. As you might expect, adolescents who have both disorders at once may display a complex mixture of attitudes and behaviors.

- Substance abuse—Adolescents with bipolar disorder are also at high risk for substance abuse. Those who have no history of preteen emotional or behavioral problems, and whose symptoms appear rather suddenly during the teen years, may be especially likely to be abusing alcohol or other drugs. At this age, illicit substances are often readily available from friends. Many adolescents with bipolar disorder, like their adult counterparts, may turn to alcohol or drugs in an attempt to smooth out their mood swings or self-treat their insomnia. Of course, substance abuse creates many problems over the long haul, and, at some point, full-fledged addiction may set in.

- Oppositional defiant disorder—This disorder is characterized by a long-lasting pattern of defiance, uncooperativeness, and hostility toward authority figures, including parents. Adolescents with either bipolar disorder or oppositional defiant disorder can appear quite irritable, surly, aggressive, and prone to temper tantrums. In addition, the grandiose beliefs of mania often look a lot like defiance to adults, since manic teenagers who are convinced of their own superior abilities or superhuman powers may not feel as if they need to listen to anyone else. As with ADHD and conduct disorder, getting a correct diagnosis depends on finding an experienced professional who can tell whether the problem is really bipolar disorder, oppositional defiant disorder, or both.

## What Is the Outlook for the Future?

Adults with bipolar disorder are more likely than children and young adolescents to have discrete periods of illness punctuated by periods of partial or complete recovery. Most adults who don't get treatment go on to have at least 10 mood episodes over the course of a lifetime. These episodes tend to become more frequent as times passes, until about the fourth or fifth episode, when the length of time between periods of illness often starts to stabilize. A single bout of untreated mania typically lasts anywhere from a few weeks to several months, and bouts of major depression may hang on even longer. It can all add up to a lot of time lost to the disease.

Compared to adults, adolescents are more likely to have prolonged or continuous symptoms, often experiencing a mixture of mania and depression at once. They also have a higher likelihood of psychotic symptoms as well as concurrent behavioral or substance abuse problems. All of these characteristics may be predictive of relatively severe illness.

However, the situation isn't as dire as it might sound. Appropriate treatment can reduce current symptoms, and, if continued long-term, may also help prevent future recurrences. It's not clear exactly how long treatment needs to be sustained for the best results, but research suggests that at least 18 months is probably the minimum, and some people may need to stay on medication for the rest of their lives. No one wants to take a medicine long-term, especially if it causes side effects. However, the potential payoff can be well worth it. The benefits of proper treatment include decreased symptoms, better functioning, and healthier psychological development during the teen years as well as less impairment farther down the road.

If you suspect that your adolescent son or daughter may be suffering from bipolar disorder, now is the time to consult a qualified professional for advice. The sooner you seek help, the better the outcome is apt to be. It's always upsetting to discover that your child has a serious illness, but there's some comfort in knowing that the steps you take now can have a positive impact on your child's future. "A few years ago, I thought the chances that

> *The sooner you seek help, the better the outcome is apt to be.*

Mike would attend college were remote," says the father of a 19-year-old with bipolar disorder. Mike was first hospitalized at age 11, and the next several years were tumultuous at best. "Yet here he is, and he's not only attending college, but he's also living away from home and doing fine." This father credits his son's progress partly to maturation—"as he's gotten more mature, he's gotten better at handling his illness"—and partly to the treatment his son has received.

## The Dangers of Doing Nothing

No matter how well your brain understands the value of prompt action, your heart may be tugging just as powerfully in the opposite direction. Denial and self-deception can be awfully tempting, especially when facing the truth means accepting that your child has a mental disorder. As the educated, professional parents of a bipolar daughter put it: "One day, our daughter experienced a major meltdown rage, where she literally ripped apart the house, screaming and yelling. So we set up an appointment for therapy, and as soon as they saw her, they quickly recognized the symptoms and told us what it was. But of course, being parents, we didn't believe them."

This is one time when it's vital not to let your emotions win the tug-of-war. As already noted, the course of depression or bipolar disorder can depend on how promptly and appropriately the disease is treated. In addition, there are a number of less obvious risks to taking a wait-and-see approach. For example, adolescents with mood disorders often have trouble in school. The longer symptoms continue, the farther behind these students are apt to fall. When depressed, they may lack sufficient motivation and energy to do their best. When manic, they may lack the focus to study or the ability to sit still and follow rules in a classroom.

> *This is one time when it's vital not to let your emotions win the tug-of-war.*

Adolescents who are depressed or manic sometimes get involved in antisocial or risk-taking behavior. Some of their actions—such as using illegal drugs, shoplifting, or vandalism—can land them in trouble with the law. One study of more than 1,800 detainees at the Cook County (Illinois) Juvenile Temporary Detention Center found that 28% of the girls and 19% of the boys met the criteria for major depression, dysthymia, or mania within the last 6 months. Of course, risky behavior, such as reckless driving, can lead to accidents as well. This is a particular concern in adolescents, for whom accidental injury is the leading cause of death.

In addition, adolescents with mood disorders may make sexual decisions that they later regret. There are several reasons for their risky sexual behavior. For one thing, they may have difficulty forming more age-appropriate relationships with peers. Their judgment and impulse control may also be impaired, and those with mania are especially prone to high-risk pleasure seeking. Add to that the substance abuse that often goes along with mood disorders, and you have a recipe for unprotected sex, teenage pregnancy, and sexually transmitted disease.

As adolescents with mood disorders grow up, some have difficulty making a smooth transition to adulthood. For example, one study from New Zealand found that adolescents who had been depressed between the ages of 14 and 16 were less likely than their nondepressed peers to have entered college by age 21. They also had a higher rate of repeated unemployment and early parenthood. In part, however, the prevalence of adult problems may reflect the fact that most adolescents with mood disorders aren't diagnosed and treated right away.

Finally, mood disorders can play a major role in the development, progression, and outcome of many medical illnesses. For example, both major depression and bipolar disorder are associated with an increased risk of death from coronary heart disease. Depression is also a consequence of many other medical conditions, including stroke, HIV/AIDS, cancer, epilepsy, obesity, and chronic pain. Research has shown that the health care costs for medical patients with major depression are about 50% higher than those for nondepressed patients.

## What Is the Risk of Suicide?

For the parents of adolescents with mood disorders, the biggest fear of all may be suicide. There is legitimate cause for concern. Suicide is the third leading cause of death among Americans ages 10 to 24, leading to the loss of more than 4,200 young lives each year. Over 90% of suicide victims have a psychiatric illness at the time of their death, and mood disorders are among the main culprits. All too often, the disorders had gone undiagnosed or untreated.

Many suicides in young people seem to be impulsive acts triggered by a stressful event, such as getting into trouble at school or with the law, breaking up with a girlfriend or boyfriend, or having a fight with friends. These events might not be sufficient in themselves to cause suicidal behavior, but when the stress is compounded by untreated depression or mania, the results can be tragic. In fact, mood disorders play a role in about two-thirds of completed suicides.

Among older teenagers, boys are about four times as likely as girls to die by suicide, but girls are twice as likely to make a suicide attempt. Death by suicide in teenagers is most often from firearms, suffocation (usually by hanging), and poisoning, in that order. Up to half of those who ultimately die by suicide have made previous attempts, which underscores the importance of taking any suicidal talk or behavior very seriously. In fact, most deaths from suicide are preceded by definite warning signs that survivors may see in retrospect, although family and friends often did not understand the urgency of the situation at the time.

As grim as these facts may be, however, it's also worth noting that suicide rates among adolescents have actually declined over the last decade. Although the reasons for this drop still aren't fully understood, it seems likely that improved recognition, diagnosis, and treatment of mood disorders played a significant role. The fact is, most adolescents who are suicidal desperately want to live but are simply unable to see another way out of their deep distress. Treatment can provide them with a life-affirming means of working toward getting well.

### What Warning Signs Should You Watch For?

Along with other signs of depression or mania, watch for these red flags that may signal suicidal thoughts or feelings in an adolescent:

- Withdrawal from friends, family, and activities
- Violent actions, rebellious behavior, or running away
- Drug or alcohol abuse
- Unusual neglect of his or her appearance
- Inability to tolerate praise or reward
- Describing himself or herself as a bad person
- Making statements such as "Nothing matters anymore," "I won't be a problem much longer," or "You won't see me again"
- Giving away prized possessions, throwing out important belongings, or otherwise putting his or her affairs in order
- Becoming cheerful overnight after a period of depression
- Having hallucinations or bizarre thoughts

If you see some of these signs in your adolescent, or if you have any reason to believe that he or she may be contemplating suicide, get help immediately. For more information on handling your teen's suicidal thoughts and feelings, see Chapter 3 (p. 98).

## The Meaning of Mental Illness

Technically speaking, a mental illness is nothing more than a mental disorder that is characterized by abnormalities in mood, emotion, thought, or higher-order behaviors, such as social interaction or the planning of future activities. It's really no different from any other medical illness that is based in one part of the body but has implications for the person as a whole. Hypertension is based in the blood vessels, asthma is based in the lungs, arthritis is based in the joints—and mental illness is based in the brain. It's a disease like any other, not a sign of poor character or evidence of a bad upbringing.

As just another disease, there should be no particular stigma attached to a mental illness such as depression or bipolar disorder. Unfortunately, that's not always the case in the real world. An adolescent who is labeled as mentally ill or emotionally disturbed (the term often used in special education) may sometimes be teased and harassed by peers, and you as the parent may sometimes be subjected to harsh criticism and finger-pointing. In recent years, however, society has slowly but surely started to become more educated about mental illness. You can hasten that education process by gently setting people straight when they make uninformed or hurtful comments about your teen's disorder.

Your willingness to talk about mental illness also sends a message of acceptance to your teenager that may translate into improved self-esteem. "Jason still doesn't like the term 'mental illness,' but he'll talk about being 'bipolar,'" says the mother of a 14-year-old. "I talk about it, too. The way I see it, it's like being born with any other illness. He can't help it, and I don't want him to be ashamed of it. It's a big part of what makes him who he is, and not necessarily in a negative way."

Mental illness, like physical illness, exists along a continuum. On one end lies mental health, in which people are able to process their thoughts and feelings in a way that leads to optimal quality of life. Mentally healthy individuals are productive at school or work, have fulfilling relationships with other people, and are able to adapt well to change and cope effectively with adversity. On the other end of the scale is mental illness, in which people have difficulty processing their thoughts and feelings, leading to emotional distress and impaired functioning.

*You can help your teen with depression or bipolar disorder move closer to the healthy end of the continuum.*

The vast majority of us exist somewhere between the two extremes, and it's hard to say exactly where the cutoff line between health and illness falls. You can help your teen with depression or bipolar disorder move closer to the healthy end of the continuum, however, by learning how to better manage his or her symptoms at home. Along the way, you'll also need to learn how to work with the school, communicate with your teen and other people in his or her life, handle the stress on your other relationships, and get professional help whenever it's necessary. You may have a long road ahead, but this book can help guide you in your journey.

## Chapter Three

# Getting the Best Treatment for Your Teen: Medications, Therapy, and More

If you're like many parents, finally getting a diagnosis of depression or bipolar disorder for your adolescent may have brought a sigh of relief. While it's not exactly good news, it *is* a name to put to the problem, and with that name often comes renewed hope for a solution. Your hope is well placed, since mood disorders are among the most treatable of all mental illnesses. Nevertheless, you've got your work cut out for you as a parent. You'll have many decisions to make and probably obstacles to overcome as you go about the business of getting help for your adolescent.

The two primary treatment options are medications and psychotherapy (the formal term for "talk therapy"). Each has been shown to be helpful for adolescents with depression and bipolar disorder. The one-two punch delivered by a combination of both may be the optimal treatment approach. For example, one study of 439 depressed adolescents between the ages of 12 and 17 looked at the combination of an antidepressant and cognitive-behavioral therapy (CBT), a popular form of psychotherapy. The researchers found that 71% of those in the study responded positively to the combination. That percentage is significantly higher than the percentage who responded to either treatment by itself (61% for medication alone and 43% for CBT alone) or to a placebo (35%). While results such as these are encouraging, it's easy to see that the first type of medication or therapy that's tried may not always do the trick. In this study, for instance, even the combination treatment failed to work for more than one-quarter of the adolescents.

To complicate matters further, the medication used in this study was fluoxetine (Prozac), which is one of several antidepressants that have recently been at the center of a scientific controversy. Concerns have been raised that these antidepressants might actually lead to suicidal thoughts and behavior in some children and teenagers. Of course, this possible risk must be weighed against the known risks of untreated depression, itself a major cause of suicide in individuals of all ages. For parents, reading headlines about the controversy can be unsettling, to say the least. The situation is only made more confusing by some news accounts, which seem more focused on exploiting the emotions aroused by youth suicide than on examining the facts.

## Your Role in the Treatment Process

As a parent, it's important to make treatment decisions for your child based on reason rather than fear. Perhaps the key fact to keep in mind is that there's no such thing as a one-size-fits-all treatment approach. If your teen shows signs of depression or bipolar disorder, your first step is to seek help promptly from a qualified mental health professional. That isn't the end of your job, however. Once you've found a doctor or therapist, you need to sit down and talk about the treatment options available for your teen, including the expected benefits and risks of each. "Don't be afraid to ask what might sound like simple questions," says one parent. And once a treatment has been prescribed, you need to keep an eye on your teen's compliance and let the treatment provider know about the results, including any adverse effects.

Science is always evolving, and the risk-benefit equation for any particular individual may change over time as new information comes to light. This is especially true of adolescents, since until recently there have been relatively few studies testing the safety and effectiveness of various treatments in teenagers. As a result, treatment providers have been forced to make judgments based on studies in adults, which may not always be applicable to younger people who are still developing, physically and psychologically. Fortunately, this is slowly but surely starting to change, as more treatments are finally being studied specifically in adolescents.

Just as your teen's treatment provider needs to stay up-to-date on the latest findings and newest treatments, you need to stay apprised of current developments, too. Reading this book or having a first discussion with the provider is only a start. As a parent, the process of learning about treatment issues is not so much a onetime undertaking as a long-term commitment.

Others who have already signed on for this commitment say the payoff is well worth the effort. In the words of a father of two teenagers, one with depression and one with bipolar disorder: "My advice to other parents? Do everything you possibly can do to get the best care for your children. You've got to fight as hard as you would if they'd fallen off a boat and you were trying to rescue them from drowning. It's that serious. The difference between good treatment, so-so treatment, and incompetent treatment can be a life-and-death issue with these kids."

"Do everything you possibly can do to get the best care for your children."

**Phases of Treatment**

Treatment for depression or bipolar disorder falls into three phases, each of which has its own distinct set of therapeutic goals.

| Phase | Goal |
| --- | --- |
| Acute | Achieve remission (a return to the level of functioning that existed before the illness) |
| Continuation | Prevent relapse (the re-emergence of symptoms) |
| Maintenance | Prevent recurrence (another episode of the illness) |

## Treatment of Depression

Depression is a serious illness that demands serious attention. It requires a treatment plan that's individualized to meet your teen's unique needs. A comprehensive plan includes psychotherapy and education about the disease. Antidepressant medications are sometimes prescribed as well, based on factors such as the severity and persistence of the symptoms and the risk of a recurrence. No two teens are exactly alike, however. For some, antidepressants may literally be lifesavers. For others, though, the risk of side effects may outweigh the potential benefits.

*If you aren't sure why your teen's treatment provider is recommending one approach over another, ask.*

A decision about which treatment approach is right for your adolescent should be based on a careful weighing of the pros and cons of all the options. If you aren't sure why your teen's treatment provider is recommending one approach over another, ask. The provider should be willing to explain why he or she believes that this course of action is the best one, on balance, for your child.

## What Types of Medication Are Used
## to Treat Depression?

Depression is rooted in a chemical imbalance within the brain, and antidepressant medications attempt to correct that imbalance. For adults with depression, several types of antidepressant have proven to be generally safe and effective. Unfortunately, much less is known about how well these drugs may work in adolescents. In fact, only one class of antidepressant—the selective serotonin reuptake inhibitors (SSRIs)—has been shown to be effective in large, well-controlled studies involving children and teens.

SSRIs—which include drugs such as fluoxetine (Prozac), paroxetine (Paxil), and sertraline (Zoloft)—are now usually the first medications tried for major depression. Although only Prozac has been specifically approved for treating depression in children and adolescents, other drugs in the class are often prescribed for young people as well. As their name implies, SSRIs work by blocking the reuptake of a brain chemical called serotonin. In other words, they interfere with the reabsorption of this chemical by the brain cells that first released it. This, in turn, increases the amount of serotonin that is available for use by the brain. SSRIs also seem to change the number and sensitivity of the brain's serotonin receptors.

SSRIs first appeared on the scene in the 1980s, and Prozac, the earliest of these drugs, became something of an overnight sensation. It was indeed a big advance over the two older types of antidepressants: tricyclic antidepressants (TCAs) and monoamine oxidase inhibitors (MAOIs). Although TCAs and SSRIs are about equally effective in adults, SSRIs tend to have less bothersome side effects. And although MAOIs may help some adults who don't respond to other antidepressants, people tak-

**Antidepressants**

Following is a list of antidepressants. MAOIs are rarely prescribed for young people because of the dietary restrictions they require.

| Type of antidepressant | Generic name | Usual brand name |
|---|---|---|
| Selective serotonin reuptake inhibitors (SSRIs) | Citalopram | Celexa |
| | Escitalopram | Lexapro |
| | Fluoxetine | Prozac |
| | Fluvoxamine | Luvox |
| | Paroxetine | Paxil |
| | Sertraline | Zoloft |
| Newer antidepressants | Bupropion | Wellbutrin |
| | Duloxetine | Cymbalta |
| | Mirtazapine | Remeron |
| | Venlafaxine | Effexor |
| Tricyclic antidepressants (TCAs) | Amitriptyline | Elavil |
| | Clomipramine | Anafranil |
| | Desipramine | Norpramin |
| | Doxepin | Sinequan |
| | Imipramine | Tofranil |
| | Maprotiline | Ludiomil |
| | Nortriptyline | Pamelor |
| | Protriptyline | Vivactil |
| | Trimipramine | Surmontil |
| Monoamine oxidase inhibitors (MAOIs) | Isocarboxazid | Marplan |
| | Phenelzine | Nardil |
| | Tranylcypromine | Parnate |

ing them have to adhere to a strictly limited diet. Such restrictions aren't necessary with SSRIs.

SSRIs soon became the best studied and most widely prescribed type of antidepressant. They are no longer the newest kids on the block, however. Since the late 1990s, several newer antidepressants have been introduced. Some—such as bupropion (Wellbutrin) and mirtazapine (Remeron)—are chemically unrelated to either SSRIs or older antidepressants. Two others— venlafaxine (Effexor) and duloxetine (Cymbalta)—inhibit the reuptake of serotonin the way SSRIs do, but also slow the reuptake of another brain chemical called norepinephrine. As a group, these newer antidepressants show promise as safe, effective drugs. Many doctors are still inclined to prescribe SSRIs first, though, because there's more research to show their effectiveness.

Today, there's an urgent need for more research to clarify the benefits and risks of all kinds of antidepressants in children and adolescents. Until more is known, it's especially critical to find a physician for your teen who is experienced with psychiatric medications. Typically, this physician would be a psychiatrist—a medical doctor who specializes in the diagnosis and treatment of mental illnesses and emotional problems. But other physicians—for example, your teen's pediatrician—and some psychiatric nurses with advanced training can prescribe medications as well.

## What Are the Benefits and Risks of SSRIs and Newer Antidepressants?

It's estimated that 11 million children and adolescents were prescribed antidepressants in 2002. A large body of evidence now shows that SSRIs can be quite effective in adults, and a smaller number of studies indicate that they often work well for younger people, too. But like all medications, SSRIs have their drawbacks. For one thing, they aren't effective or tolerable for everyone with depression. Adults who don't do well on SSRIs can turn to the other types of antidepressants. For adolescents, however, the situation is more problematic, since there's a dearth of hard evidence to show that the other classes of antidepressants are actually safe and effective in young people.

SSRIs also may cause side effects, including headache and nausea. Problems with sexual functioning are fairly common in both males and females. In addition, some people who take SSRIs experience anxiety, panic attacks, agitation, trouble sleeping, irritability, hostility, impulsiveness, or extreme restlessness. It has been suggested that people who develop these symptoms early in their treatment might be at risk for sinking deeper into depression or becoming suicidal, although this link has yet to be proven.

Since it's much better to be safe than sorry, though, contact the doctor promptly if these symptoms develop or worsen after your teen starts an SSRI. As one parent puts it, "You need to understand how important you are to the process. The psychiatrist isn't there with your child 24/7. He's not seeing the effects of the meds. Don't be afraid to call him back if you see anything that doesn't make sense to you."

*"You need to understand how important you are to the process."*

The newer antidepressants seem to work at least as well as SSRIs in adults. Each newer antidepressant has its own set of side effects, but many of the common ones are similar to those of SSRIs. Wellbutrin may also in rare cases cause seizures or psychosis in people who are predisposed to those problems. As with SSRIs, parents should be alert for any increased jitteriness, agitation, or insomnia in teens taking these drugs.

---

### Red Flags

If your teen starts taking an antidepressant, let the doctor know promptly if these symptoms develop or grow worse:

- anxiety • panic attacks • agitation • irritability • hostility
- impulsiveness • extreme restlessness • insomnia
- self-injurious behavior • suicidal thoughts

## Do Antidepressants Increase the Risk of Suicide?

Of all the potential side effects of antidepressants, by far the most worrisome is their possible association with suicidal thoughts or behavior. The drugs that have been directly implicated in this regard are SSRIs and newer antidepressants—in other words, the medications that are most frequently prescribed. The relationship between the use of these antidepressants and the risk of suicide remains unclear, however. It's an extremely difficult issue to study, because suicide is already a significant risk among those who are depressed. In fact, some experts have pointed out that the rise in SSRI use has actually coincided with a fall in suicide rates among adolescents. It seems logical that this might be partly due to better treatment of depression with SSRIs and newer antidepressants, but that connection is still speculative.

At the same time, a growing number of reports have surfaced that a small percentage of individuals of all ages may become suicidal after starting antidepressant treatment. In September 2004, the U.S. Food and Drug Administration (FDA) held a hearing specifically on the risk of suicide among children and adolescents who are taking antidepressants. In a combined analysis of 24 studies involving over 4,400 young people with major depression and other mental disorders, the FDA found not a single death from suicide. Nevertheless, it did find an increased risk of suicidal thinking or behavior during the first few months of treatment with antidepressants. The average risk of suicidal thinking or behavior was 4% in young people taking an antidepressant, compared to 2% in young people taking a placebo.

The risk seemed to apply to every antidepressant that had been studied in placebo-controlled trials involving children or

## FDA Warning

In October 2004, the FDA directed makers of all antidepressant drugs to add stronger warning statements to their product labeling. The FDA determined that the following points are appropriate for inclusion in the warning:

- Antidepressants increase the risk of suicidal thinking and behavior (suicidality) in children and adolescents with major depression and other mental disorders.
- Health care professionals considering the use of an antidepressant in a child or adolescent for any clinical purpose must balance the risk of increased suicidality with the clinical need.
- Patients who are started on therapy should be observed closely for clinical worsening, suicidality, or unusual changes in behavior.
- Families and caregivers should be advised to closely observe the patient and to communicate with the prescriber.
- A statement regarding whether the particular drug is approved for any pediatric indications and, if so, which ones. (Only Prozac has been specifically approved for the treatment of major depression in pediatric patients. Prozac, Zoloft, Luvox, and Anafranil are approved for treating pediatric obsessive-compulsive disorder, a type of anxiety disorder.)

For the latest information, see the FDA website at www.fda.gov.

adolescents. The drugs that fell into this category were all SSRIs or newer antidepressants, mainly because they're the medications that are still the subject of active research. However, members of an FDA advisory committee recommended that any new warning about the risk of suicide in young people be applied across the board to *all* antidepressants. They reasoned that the suicide risk might not be as apparent with other drugs simply because they aren't used as often and haven't been studied in young people.

In October 2004, the FDA responded by directing drug companies to add stronger warning statements to the health professional labeling of all antidepressant medications. The FDA also decided that written material for patients and families about antidepressant risks and precautions should be handed out by pharmacists with new prescriptions or refills of any antidepressant.

But as important as it is to consider the suicide risk, it's also critical to keep that risk in perspective. Many of the experts testifying at the FDA hearing stressed the value of antidepressants for young people who are dangerously depressed and out of other options. Speaking at the hearing on behalf of the American Psychiatric Association, Dr. David Fassler summed it up this way: "Every suicide is a tragedy, and any increased risk of suicidal thoughts or behaviors, no matter how small, must be taken very seriously. However, based on the data currently available, most clinicians believe, and I would concur, that for children and adolescents who suffer from depression, the potential benefit of these medications far outweighs the risk."

> . . . as important as it is to consider the suicide risk, it's also critical to keep that risk in perspective.

### Who Is Most Likely to Be Helped by Antidepressants?

Clearly, antidepressants are powerful medicine, and the decision to give them to an adolescent should be based on careful consideration. For those who truly need them, however, antidepressants may be invaluable weapons in the treatment arsenal. At present, antidepressants are still often the first-choice treatment for young people with moderate to severe symptoms who are unable to participate fully in psychotherapy. Antidepressants are also frequently prescribed for teenagers with long-lasting or recurring episodes of depression as well as those who have tried psychotherapy but found that it didn't provide enough relief by itself.

*Antidepressants may be invaluable weapons in the treatment arsenal.*

One catch, though, is that antidepressants may sometimes trigger a first episode of mania in people who have bipolar disorder, but whose illness starts out with depression. Antidepressants may also cause more rapid cycling of moods in people with bipolar disorder. These are some of the risks your teen's doctor will take into account when deciding whether to prescribe an antidepressant. To assess whether your teen's depression is actually the first manifestation of bipolar disorder, the doctor will probably ask questions about your teen's symptoms and your family history of mood disorders.

The possibility that an antidepressant might lead to switching—the rapid transition from depression to mania—is something about which parents should be forewarned. Unfortunately, some aren't, and the sudden switch in mood catches them off guard. Roberta is a master's-level nurse who teaches at the nursing school of a university, but even she had never heard about switching until her son went through it:

> "We took him to a psychiatrist in the first place because he was just staying in his room all the time," Roberta says. "He wouldn't go to school, wouldn't see his friends. It was like the whole world was dark for him. When the psychiatrist put him on Paxil, he was instantly better. He was out of his room and hanging out with his friends. But then, boom!—all of a sudden, he was everywhere at once."
>
> By the time Roberta realized what was happening, her son had slipped into a severely manic state that required him to be sedated for a while. Because she was a nurse, Roberta was able to take a three-month medical leave and care for him at home. But it was a harrowing experience for both of them, and she wishes she had been told to watch for the warning signs of impending mania.

## What's the Bottom Line on Medications for Depression?

To be on the safe side, any adolescent who is taking an antidepressant should be under the care of a physician with expertise in psychiatric medications. Special attention should be paid to the first few weeks after the antidepressant is started, since this is when any untoward side effects are most likely to appear. Once your teen starts an antidepressant, let the doctor know promptly if you notice new signs of nervousness, agitation, insomnia, irritability, mood swings, suicidal talk or behavior, or worsening depression.

Don't expect a dramatic turnaround in your teen's mood overnight. With an SSRI, for instance, it can take 4 to 6 weeks for the full effects to be felt. If your teen still isn't feeling any better after that time, the doctor may try increasing the dose, changing to another drug, or adding a second medication. Since there is no way to know in advance how a particular person will react to a given antidepressant, some trial and error may be required to find the best medication and dosage.

Once an effective treatment has been found, it's usually continued for 6 to 12 months, and sometimes longer, to decrease the chances of a relapse or recurrence. After your teen's depression has lifted, it can be tempting to stop the medication right away. But if you do this too soon or too abruptly, the depression may return. Occasionally, people also develop discontinuation symptoms if they stop an antidepressant too suddenly. When the time comes for your teen to stop the drug, the doctor may advise you to taper it off gradually over several weeks.

Few parents like the idea of giving any potent medication to their adolescents. For many, however, the bottom line is that antidepressants may be able to break through a teen's dark mood

## Do Ask, Do Tell

If medication is part of your teen's treatment plan, be sure to tell the doctor about any other medications, over-the-counter drugs, or herbal supplements your teen is taking, since some drugs interact harmfully with each other. Let the doctor know about any drug allergies your teen has as well. Then make sure you have all the facts you need about any new medication that is prescribed. Here are some questions you may want to ask:

- What are the generic and brand names of the medication?
- What is it supposed to do?
- How soon should we see results?
- When and how often should my teen take the medication?
- How long should my teen stay on the medication?
- Will my teen need to limit any activities while taking the drug?
- Does the medication interact with alcohol, other drugs, or certain foods?
- What are the possible side effects of the medication?
- Which of these side effects are most serious?
- What should I do if these side effects occur?
- What number should I call if I have any questions or concerns?

when nothing else can. As one father of a 17-year-old put it, "Maria's on antidepressants, and, mood-wise, she's doing much better. She's still having some attendance and self-discipline problems at school. But she's getting A's and B's, and she's enjoying life again. That's *really* good to see."

## What Forms of Psychotherapy Are Used to Treat Depression?

While antidepressants address the chemical bases of depression, psychotherapy targets the psychological, social, and behavioral aspects of the illness. Interestingly, recent research using sophisticated brain imaging technology shows that psychotherapy may lead to physical changes in brain pathways as well. However, the pattern of brain changes is somewhat different from that seen in people taking antidepressants. This raises the tantalizing prospect that treatment providers might one day be able to use brain scans to prescribe the exact type of psychotherapy and/or medication that's best for targeting the precise cause of an individual's depression.

For now, though, providers must rely on treatments that have shown in studies to work in many of the people, much of the time. Psychotherapy is one such treatment. While there are several schools of psychotherapy, one thing they all have in common is that the person talks with a therapist in order to gain insight into problems or learn skills for coping with daily life and managing symptoms. When it comes to the treatment of depression in adolescents, the best-studied form of psychotherapy is cognitive-behavioral therapy (CBT), which aims to correct ingrained patterns of thinking and behavior that may be contributing to the illness.

The cognitive part of CBT helps people identify unrealistically negative thoughts and habitually pessimistic attitudes. Such thoughts can then be reframed in more realistically positive or optimistic terms. The behavioral part of CBT helps people change maladaptive behaviors and learn to get more enjoyment from their everyday activities. One way this is done is by teaching people to break down large tasks into smaller, more manageable chunks. Another way is by giving people a chance to rehearse the social skills and coping strategies they need to build healthier relationships and deal with

*The behavioral part of CBT helps people change maladaptive behaviors . . .*

their illness effectively. CBT can help teens with depression learn to:

- think more positively
- monitor their moods
- schedule pleasant activities
- set and achieve goals
- cope with social situations
- relax and manage stress
- solve many everyday problems

Interpersonal psychotherapy (IPT) is another approach that has proven effective against depression in adults. Although less research has been done in young people with depression, the evidence to date looks promising for them as well. The idea behind IPT is that, although depression may be caused by a number of factors, the immediate trigger is usually an interpersonal problem. This problem typically involves grief over a recent loss, a change in social role, the lack of social skills, or a dispute with another person. IPT helps an individual first identify the problem that triggered the current episode of depression, then develop the necessary social and communication skills to resolve the problem effectively. IPT can help teens with depression learn to handle social issues such as:

- coping with parental divorce or separation
- establishing their independence
- dealing with peer pressure
- forming healthy friendships
- resolving family conflicts

Either CBT or IPT may be used in individual therapy, in which a person works one-on-one with a therapist. However, these approaches are also used in settings where more than one person meets with a therapist at the same time. Family therapy is one example. It involves bringing several members of a family together for therapy sessions. Family therapy helps families work together to identify and change the destructive patterns that may contribute to or arise from a teen's depression. This kind of therapy can uncover hidden issues, such as the resentment a sibling may feel because of all the attention the depressed teen is getting. It can also open lines of communication and teach everyone coping skills for dealing with the teen's illness. Other possible goals of family therapy include strengthening family bonds, reducing conflict in the home, and improving empathy among family members.

Group therapy gives adolescents with depression a chance to trade concerns and insights with other teens who are struggling with similar issues. Under the guidance of the therapist leading the group, members can benefit from each other's emotional support and practical advice. The group setting also offers teens a chance to learn and practice social skills. In addition, the discussion of shared experiences helps depressed adolescents realize that they aren't alone in their problems and

*Other teens have battled the same demons, and many have won.*

anxieties. Other teens have battled the same demons, and many have won. This message can be a powerful antidote to feelings of helplessness and hopelessness.

### What Are the Benefits and Risks of Psychotherapy?

All of these forms of psychotherapy are intended to help people address the emotional, cognitive, behavioral, and social problems associated with depression. There is good evidence that psychotherapy in general, and CBT in particular, can indeed help in this regard. More than a dozen randomized controlled trials—the gold standard in clinical research—have now looked at CBT for young people with depression. Taken as a whole, these trials have found that CBT was more effective than either no treatment or a control condition in which the participants got extra attention without formal therapy. This effectiveness held up in a wide range of treatment formats, including both individual and group therapy with a varying number of sessions.

Less research has been done on IPT and family therapy in depressed adolescents, but the results so far are encouraging. In one head-to-head comparison, IPT seemed to be at least as effective as CBT. In another study, family therapy that focused on repairing and strengthening the emotional bonds among family members seemed to get results that were as good as either CBT or IPT.

Many of these studies have been conducted in the rarefied world of university-based facilities with ample resources and highly trained therapists. Unfortunately, most adolescents in the real world don't have access to these kinds of treatment opportunities. That's why it's especially heartening when studies done under more typical conditions also get positive results. A case in point is a study conducted at five school-based mental health clinics in low-income neighborhoods of New York City. The study included 63 students, ages 12 to 18, with some type of depressive disorder. Half were assigned to get 16 weeks of IPT provided by the schools' regular social workers or psychologists, none of whom had previous experience with this type of therapy before being trained for the study. The other half got the usual treatment offered by the school clinics. Students in the IPT group showed a greater decrease in symptoms and more improvement in overall functioning, demonstrating that this kind of structured therapy can get good results even under less-than-ideal circumstances.

Unlike medication, psychotherapy doesn't have the same potential for causing adverse physical reactions. Nevertheless, it's not entirely risk-free. By its very nature, psychotherapy often taps into deep, and sometimes disturbing, thoughts and feelings. It's essential that a therapist be prepared to handle any unexpected reactions that might arise. If your adolescent is taking medication, the therapist should be knowledgeable about the effects of these drugs and willing to coordinate treatment with your teen's psychiatrist or other physician. If your teen has other mental, emotional, or behavioral disorders in addition to depression, the therapist should be well versed in these conditions as well.

## Who Is Most Likely to Be Helped by Psychotherapy?

Psychotherapy is sometimes used alone for the treatment of milder depression. When depression is moderate to severe, psychotherapy is often combined with medication. Providers include psychiatrists, clinical psychologists, clinical social workers, mental health counselors, psychiatric nurses, and marriage and family therapists. When selecting a therapist for your adolescent, factors to consider include the person's training and experience, his or her expertise in working with young people, your comfort level with the therapist, and the therapeutic approach that is employed.

For the best results, your adolescent should be willing and able to work together with the therapist in a spirit of trust, honesty, and cooperation. In CBT and sometimes in other types of psychotherapy, the therapist may assign homework. For example, the therapist may ask your teen to keep a journal or practice new skills. To get the most out of therapy, it's helpful if your teen does the homework regularly.

*The therapist may ask your teen to keep a journal or practice new skills.*

## What's the Bottom Line on Psychotherapy for Depression?

As an initial treatment for milder depression, psychotherapy can help adolescents develop critical social skills and coping strategies. It can also help families manage the interpersonal conflict that is often associated with the illness. When combined with medication for more severe depression, psychotherapy can help teens address the emotional, cognitive, behavioral, and social aspects of their disease. The likelihood that depression will recur after CBT is higher for teens who start out with more severe symptoms or who come from families with serious discord. Therefore, a combination of treatments may be especially important to prevent a recurrence in such teens.

In studies of CBT, good results have generally been achieved in anywhere from 5 to 16 sessions. The exact number of sessions needed for a particular adolescent depends on many factors, including the nature and severity of the symptoms. Unfortunately, the amount of time your teen spends in therapy may also be dictated to some extent by the terms of your insurance coverage.

At first, psychotherapy sessions may be scheduled weekly. But as your teen starts to get better, the sessions may gradually be spaced farther apart. Even after your teen's symptoms have improved, it's often helpful if less frequent sessions are continued for several months. Continuing psychotherapy provides teens and families with a chance to keep practicing and consolidating the skills they learned earlier in the therapy process. It also gives teens an opportunity to solidify their understanding of the thoughts and behaviors that might otherwise contribute to a relapse.

At some point during the first few sessions, your adolescent and the therapist will usually work together to create a list of short-term and long-term goals. It's a good idea to revisit this list periodically to see whether progress is being made. As with medication, though, it's essential to give psychotherapy enough time to work. If you expect instant results, you're apt to be disappointed. On the other hand, it's reasonable to expect gradual but noticeable progress over a period of time. Your teenager's therapist may be able to give you some idea of how soon your teen is likely to start noticing improvement and how long therapy is expected to last.

This is just an estimate, and the timetable may need to be adjusted as the therapist learns more about your teen's individual response to the treatment. If therapy is taking much longer than planned, however, feel free to ask the therapist why. You'll probably wind up with a much clearer picture of your teen's situation. If you get an evasive or unsatisfactory answer, you might consider seeking a second opinion, just as you would for any other illness.

### What Is Light Therapy?

Light therapy—also called phototherapy—involves a regimen of daily exposure to very bright light from an artificial source. The intensity of the light is similar to that of early morning sunlight and many times brighter than that of normal indoor light fixtures. Light therapy is sometimes used as a treatment for seasonal affective disorder (SAD), a pattern of seasonal depression that typically starts in fall or winter and subsides in the spring. While many people develop a mild case of the winter doldrums, those with SAD sink into full-fledged major depression. This reaction is thought to be linked to the shorter days and reduced exposure to sunlight in winter.

The exact biological mechanisms that cause SAD are still uncertain. However, it's known that light exposure affects the brain's production of a hormone called melatonin. This hormone regulates the body's internal clock, which controls daily rhythms of sleep, body temperature, and hormone secretion. Melatonin is produced by the brain during periods of darkness. Winter's short, gloomy days and long, dark nights set the stage for greater production of this hormone. One theory is that an overabundance of melatonin may trigger depressive symptoms in some individuals. Another theory suggests that light may alter the activity of certain neurotransmitters, such as serotonin and dopamine, that are also involved in other forms of depression.

Whatever the explanation, research has found that exposure to intense artificial light may relieve the symptoms of SAD for many adults. In studies with adults, over half of light therapy users show nearly complete remission of symptoms, although the treatment must be continued throughout the entire season to maintain this improvement. But a word of caution: Light therapy has not been well studied in children and adolescents, so it's not known if the treatment works as well for young people.

Typically, the treatment consists of sitting in front of a special light box that contains fluorescent bulbs or tubes covered by a plastic screen. The box is positioned so that light enters a person's eyes indirectly, and the screen helps block out potentially harmful ultraviolet rays. Users should be cautioned not to look straight at the box, though, because the intense light could be harmful to their eyes. A typical prescription might involve gradually working up to spending 30 to 60 minutes per day in front of a light box at a designated time. The best time for the sessions is usually in the morning.

Light therapy may be the first treatment tried for milder cases of seasonal depression. For those with more severe seasonal depression, light therapy may sometimes be combined with antidepressant medications. Most people who respond to the light start to improve in a week or less, but some need several weeks to feel the full effects. Light therapy requires a time commitment, but that time can be spent reading, using a computer, watching television, or eating breakfast. Possible side effects include eyestrain, headache, and irritability. The therapy may not be appropriate for people who have light-sensitive skin, are taking a medication that reacts with sunlight, or have an eye condition that might make them especially susceptible to eye damage. Extra care must be taken by those who have a history or high risk of bipolar disorder, since light therapy might potentially trigger the switch to a manic state.

Although light boxes are widely sold without a prescription, they should be used under the guidance of an experienced doctor or therapist. They're not for everyone, but light therapy may brighten the mood of some adolescents with seasonal depression. One mother recalls, "Allie is very verbal, and she used to say things like, 'Just look at all this gray. I can feel myself getting depressed.' So her psychiatrist prescribed a light box, and it seemed to lift her mood. The cat and dog would come sit by her because they liked the light. I think it improved the cat's mood, too!"

**What Is Electroconvulsive Therapy?**

Electroconvulsive therapy (ECT) involves delivering a carefully controlled electrical current to the brain, which produces a brief seizure. This form of therapy has gotten an undeserved bad rap in the public mind. For many people, it still raises the specter of "shock therapy" and *One Flew Over the Cuckoo's Nest*. Yet ECT can be a highly effective treatment for severe mood disorders when more conservative treatments have not been successful. In fact, research indicates that at least three-quarters of those who receive ECT for mood disorders have a positive response. In a recent practice guideline, the American Academy of Child and Adolescent Psychiatry concluded that ECT may be appropriate for some adolescents with severe mood disorders when at least two medications have been tried without success or when the symptoms are so urgent that there isn't time to wait for a medication to work.

ECT is thought to act by temporarily altering some of the electrochemical processes involved in brain functioning. The person undergoing ECT is first given a muscle relaxant and general anesthesia. Electrodes are then placed at precise locations on the person's head, and the brain is stimulated by a brief, controlled series of electrical pulses. This stimulation leads to a seizure within the brain that lasts for about a minute. Thanks to the muscle relaxant, the rest of the person's body doesn't convulse. The anesthesia keeps the person from feeling any pain. A few minutes later, the person awakens, just as someone would after minor surgery.

ECT generally consists of 6 to 12 such treatments, which are typically given three times a week. The effects appear gradually over the course of ECT, although they usually are felt sooner than with medication. The most common immediate side effects are headache, muscle ache or soreness, nausea, and confusion. Such effects usually occur within hours of a treatment and generally clear up quickly. However, as the treatments go on, people also may have trouble remembering newly learned

*. . . some people report that their memory is actually better after ECT*

information. In addition, some people experience partial loss of their memories from the days, weeks, or months preceding ECT. While most of these memory problems resolve within days to months of completing the last treatment, they occasionally last longer. On the other hand, some people report that their memory is actually better after ECT, since their mind is no longer operating in a fog of depression.

### What Are Some Emerging Therapies for Depression?

The concept of stimulating the brain to alter its electrical and chemical functioning has also led to the development of newer treatment approaches that are still being tested. In vagus nerve stimulation (VNS), a small battery-powered device, similar to a pacemaker, is implanted in the left upper chest area. A thin wire inside the body connects this device to the left vagus nerve, located on the left side of the neck. This nerve, in turn, connects to parts of the brain that play a role in mood and sleep. The device is programmed to deliver mild electrical pulses at regular intervals to the vagus nerve, which then stimulates those parts of the brain. The device can also be activated by the depressed person with a special magnet. In theory, the stimulation may affect activity within the brain in a way that helps correct the biochemical processes underlying depression.

VNS was originally developed and approved by the FDA for the treatment of a certain hard-to-treat type of epilepsy. Doctors observed that many of the epilepsy patients who had a VNS device implanted not only had fewer seizures but also experienced a lift in their mood. This observation raised the possibility that the same device might be useful for treating severe depression as well. Thus far, the results of studies in adult patients with severe, long-term depression seem promising. At this writing, the company that makes the VNS device has applied for FDA approval to market it for chronic or recurrent depression in adults who have unsuccessfully tried several other forms of treatment. The FDA has not yet made a final decision on the application but has authorized the company to study the treatment of 100 individuals at multiple sites across the United States.

If VNS is ultimately approved as a depression treatment, one drawback to its use will be the possible side effects, which include hoarseness, sore throat, and shortness of breath. Other risks include complications from the surgery to implant the device, malfunctioning of the device, or dislodging of the device or wire inside the body. Clearly, this is an invasive technique that would most likely be used only as a last resort. But for the minority of people with depression who aren't helped by any type of medication or psychotherapy, the emergence of VNS seems to offer fresh hope for the future.

Other new technologies are under investigation as well. For example, transcranial magnetic stimulation (TMS) has been studied as a possible treatment for mental illness since 1995. In TMS, a special electromagnet is placed near the scalp, where it can be used to deliver short bursts of energy to stimulate the nerve cells in a specific part of the brain. The latest generation of TMS devices are capable of delivering up to 50 energy pulses per second. One advantage to this treatment is that it doesn't require surgery, hospitalization, or anesthesia. A physician simply applies the device in treatment sessions that last about 30 minutes each. Current evidence suggests that such treatments should be given 5 days per week for 2 to 4 weeks.

In studies to date, most side effects of TMS seem to be relatively mild and infrequent. They include discomfort, headache, or lightheadedness during treatment, which usually goes away soon after the session ends. There is also a chance that the treatment might trigger a seizure, but new treatment guidelines have been instituted to decrease this risk. TMS is still considered an experimental procedure, but it may one day join the ever-growing roster of treatment options for people with depression.

## Do Dietary Supplements Help With Depression?

Another approach that some people have tried is the use of dietary supplements to treat depression. One of the most popular is an herb called St. John's wort (*Hypericum perforatum*), which has been used for centuries in the treatment of mental disorders and nerve pain. In Europe, St. John's wort is currently a prescription medication for depression. In the United States, where it's sold without a prescription, St. John's wort is one of the top-selling herbal products. Research suggests that the herb may be helpful for treating very mild depression. This does not seem to be the case when the symptoms are more substantial, however. A large, carefully designed study funded by the National Institutes of Health found that St. John's wort was no more effective than a placebo for the treatment of moderate depression.

Nevertheless, many people find the notion of a "natural" remedy very appealing. But just because a substance is sold as an herbal product rather than a pharmaceutical one doesn't make it entirely risk-free. In the case of St. John's wort, the most common side effects include dry mouth, dizziness, diarrhea, nausea, fatigue, and increased sensitivity to sunlight. In addition, St. John's wort may interact with several medications, including oral contraceptives, decreasing their effectiveness. There's also a possibility that the herb may interact harmfully with certain antidepressant medications, including the widely prescribed SSRIs.

SAM-e (S-adenosyl-L-methionine, or "Sammy" for short) is a second supplement that has been touted for depression. It's a compound that occurs naturally in all living cells and is a key player in biochemical reactions within the human body. Among other things, this compound plays an important role in regulating serotonin and dopamine, two brain chemicals linked to depression. Some studies suggest that SAM-e supplements may reduce the symptoms of depression, although the results are not definitive. Common side effects include nausea and constipation.

St. John's wort and SAM-e are among the better-studied dietary supplements. Because such supplements don't have to go through the FDA approval process, however, neither has been subjected to the same rigorous scrutiny as prescription antidepressants. Perhaps the biggest risk of these products is that people will forego proven treatments for unproven remedies. If you think you might want to try a supplement with your adolescent, be sure to discuss it first with the doctor, who can evaluate whether this is a safe and sensible approach for your teen.

## Treatment of Bipolar Disorder

The mainstay of treatment for bipolar disorder is medication. The oldest and best-known such medication is lithium, an alkaline substance found in trace amounts in the human body, plants, and mineral rocks. Over 1,800 years ago, the Greek physician Galen prescribed bathing in and drinking from alkaline springs as a treatment for manic patients. Today, lithium remains widely prescribed for bipolar disorder, but it has also been joined by other mood-stabilizing medications.

These medications can be extremely valuable. Taken alone, however, they can't address all the wide-ranging psychological, social, and behavioral issues related to bipolar disorder. That's why psychotherapy also has a central role in any comprehensive treatment plan for the illness. Psychotherapy can maximize the effectiveness of drug therapy, especially when it's combined with education about the illness and necessary support services. Among other things, psycho-therapy can help teens with bipolar disorder reduce their stress, rebuild their relationships, and reinforce their self-esteem.

*Psychotherapy also has a central role in any comprehensive treatment plan for the illness.*

## What Types of Medication Are Used to Treat Bipolar Disorder?

The modern use of lithium as a psychiatric medication can be traced back to the late 1940s, when an Australian psychiatrist named John Cade was conducting experiments on guinea pigs in his lab. Cade suspected that mania in humans might be caused by excess uric acid in the body. To test this hypothesis, he decided to inject the animals with uric acid, which he administered in a solution of lithium salts. When Cade gave the guinea pigs their injections, however, he was in for a surprise. The normally active animals grew calm and impassive. Cade had stumbled upon the anti-manic effects of lithium, which eventually became the first mood stabilizer—a medication that reduces manic symptoms and helps even out mood swings.

It's still unclear exactly how lithium has this effect, although the drug is thought to help correct a chemical imbalance in the brain. One line of current research is looking at the effect of

## Mood Stabilizers

Following is a list of mood stabilizers. Also included in this list are several antipsychotic medications that are sometimes prescribed along with or instead of the standard mood-stabilizing drugs.

| Type of mood stabilizer | Generic name | Brand name |
| --- | --- | --- |
| Lithium | Lithium carbonate | Eskalith, Lithane, Lithobid |
| | Lithium citrate | Cibalith-S |
| Anticonvulsants | Carbamazepine | Tegretol |
| | Lamotrigine | Lamictal |
| | Valproic acid, divalproex sodium | Depakote |
| Atypical antipsychotics | Aripiprazole | Abilify |
| | Clozapine | Clozaril |
| | Olanzapine | Zyprexa |
| | Quetiapine | Seroquel |
| | Risperidone | Risperdal |
| | Ziprasidone | Geodon |

lithium on second messengers, molecules inside nerve cells that let certain parts of the cell know when a specific receptor has been activated by a neurotransmitter. Second messengers complete the communication process when a neurotransmitter relays a message from one cell to another. By affecting this process, lithium might influence the flow of messages within the brain. This is just one of several possible explanations for lithium's effect.

Lithium remained the standard treatment for bipolar disorder for many years, and it's still very widely prescribed today. Recently, though, doctors have come to realize that many anticonvulsants—medications that help prevent seizures—have mood-stabilizing effects as well. One such drug, called valproic acid (Depakote), has proved to be so effective that it's now often used as a first-choice treatment for bipolar disorder. In fact, a National Institute of Mental Health study that looked at the everyday medical treatment of young people with bipolar disorder found that more had been treated with Depakote than lithium.

## What Are the Benefits and Risks of Mood Stabilizers?

In adults with bipolar disorder, well-controlled studies have shown that, on average, lithium can reduce the number of both manic and depressive episodes. It doesn't work equally well for everyone, though. For some individuals, it can be quite effective. However, about 42% to 64% of adults with bipolar disorder don't respond to lithium. They may do better on an anticonvulsant.

Less research has been done on the use of mood stabilizers by adolescents. The available evidence suggests that teens probably respond to the same mood-stabilizing medications as adults. Similar to the findings with adults, studies have shown that about half of young people respond to lithium treatment, and half don't. Among those who do respond, some experience only partial improvement with lithium alone. In general, the odds of a good response to lithium are better among people with a family history of mood disorders and those whose episodes of mania and depression are punctuated by periods of relative wellness.

*. . . about half of young people respond to lithium treatment*

When lithium works, it can be invaluable. Along with the drug's benefits come some risks, however. For one thing, there is a narrow dosage range at which the medication is effective. If too little is taken, a person may not get the therapeutic effects, but if too much is taken, the drug can be toxic. Since the difference between a therapeutic dose and a toxic one is so small, close monitoring is needed to make sure that blood levels don't inadvertently rise too high. Frequent blood tests may be needed at the start of lithium therapy until the best dosage level has been determined. After that, blood levels may be checked every few months or so.

Factors such as dehydration or other medications can affect lithium levels between blood tests. Signs of lithium toxicity include nausea, vomiting, drowsiness, confusion, slurred speech, blurred vision, dizziness, muscle twitching, irregular heartbeat, and eventually seizures. This is an emergency situation, and, if not treated promptly, the symptoms can become life-threatening. If your teen develops these symptoms, get medical help immediately.

Even at therapeutic levels, lithium can cause side effects, such as drowsiness, weakness, nausea, fatigue, hand tremor, or increased thirst. Lithium can also lead to weight gain, a side effect that is troubling for many teens. In addition, the drug's effects on the kidneys may result in increased urination or bedwetting. Finally, lithium can cause the thyroid gland to become underactive or enlarged, so thyroid function tests need to be a regular part of lithium therapy. If thyroid underactivity is detected, your teen may need to take thyroid hormone pills.

Anticonvulsants are the main alternative to lithium. In the largest study of Depakote among young people with bipolar disorder, about 60% felt better with the medication. Tegretol has also been found effective in a smaller percentage of young people. One advantage to these drugs is that they aren't as toxic as lithium if a person accidentally takes too much. But like other medications, anticonvulsants can lead to side effects. For example, Depakote may cause nausea, headache, double vision, dizziness, anxiety, or confusion. Since it affects the liver, tests of liver function should be done periodically. Depakote can also cause weight gain. In addition, there is some evidence suggesting that teenage girls who take Depakote may be at risk for amenorrhea (the abnormal absence of menstruation), excess facial and body hair, and polycystic ovary syndrome (cysts in the ovaries).

Since mood stabilizers can cause significant side effects, some teens may be reluctant to take them. "My son gained weight, and he blames the medication," says the mother of a 14-year-old with bipolar disorder. "It bothers him a lot. He's already stigmatized by the illness, so it's a double whammy." If you find yourself in a similar situation, start an honest dialogue with your teen about the pros and the cons of the medication. Cooperation will come a lot easier if your teen sees how the positives of taking a drug outweigh the negatives.

> Start an honest dialogue with your teen about the pros and the cons of the medication.

## When Are Other Types of Medications Helpful?

For some people, the present episode of mania does not completely respond to a mood stabilizer alone. Or episodes of mania or depression may break through despite taking a mood stabilizer. In such cases, another type of medication may be prescribed along with the mood stabilizer to help control the symptoms. Atypical antipsychotics—drugs such as risperidone (Risperdal), olanzapine (Zyprexa), quetiapine (Seroquel), aripiprazole (Abilify), ziprasidone (Geodon), and clozapine (Clozaril)—are used to treat severe mental disorders. They may be helpful for symptoms such as hallucinations or delusions. Even in the absence of such distorted thinking, antipsychotics can sometimes help control the symptoms of bipolar disorder if a mood

## Taking Their Medicine

Finding an effective medication for your adolescent is one thing. Getting your teen to actually take it can be quite another. Teens may resist taking their medicine for several reasons, including unpleasant side effects, simple forgetfulness, and a desire to be like their friends. Below are parent-tested tips on encouraging adherence to a medication plan:

- Educate your teen so that he or she knows what to expect. "Let your child know that medication may take a few weeks to work properly. Also, it's important to tell your child not to give up hope if the first medication doesn't work. There are so many different options now."

- Encourage frank talk about medication with others who need to know. "My daughter is fairly open with her little group of friends. She takes medication at 6:00 in the morning and 6:00 at night. It's not unusual for her to be gone in the evening, or even in the morning if she's going to a slumber party, but she's good about taking her meds away from home."

- Take responsibility for storing and supervising the medication for a child under 18. "In our home, it's just known that everyone takes their medication, including me. I'm in charge of setting out all our medications at night. I put them in those little seven-day pillboxes, so we can see at a glance if anyone forgot to take their medication today."

- Set clear expectations for older adolescents who are still living at home. "Because this illness can have such a detrimental effect on the family, when my children turned 18, they were told that if they wanted to continue to live at home, they had to keep taking their medication."

stabilizer alone isn't sufficient. Possible side effects associated with atypical antipsychotics, especially Zyprexa and Clozaril, include weight gain, high blood sugar, and diabetes.

Adolescents with bipolar disorder are likely to experience depression as well as mania, so antidepressants may be prescribed, too. Great care must be taken, though, since antidepressants can trigger a switch to mania or cause more rapid cycling of moods. To protect against this, mood stabilizers are usually continued at the same time. In addition, anti-anxiety medications—such as alprazolam (Xanax) or lorazepam (Ativan)—are sometimes prescribed for short-term use to help control the nervousness, racing thoughts, and distress that may go along with mania.

## What's the Bottom Line on Medications for Bipolar Disorder?

In people who respond to lithium, the symptoms of severe mania usually start to subside within 5 to 14 days after the medication is started, but it can take weeks to months for the symptoms to be fully controlled. Antipsychotic medications are sometimes prescribed in the interim to help control the manic symptoms until the lithium begins to take hold. Once a person's mood has stabilized, lithium may be continued long-term to help prevent a relapse or recurrence. In some people, this prevents future episodes altogether, while in others, it may lessen the severity or frequency of episodes. For still others, lithium may not help at all. Unfortunately, there's no way to predict in advance who will or won't respond. The only way to know for sure is to give the medication a trial and carefully monitor the outcome.

Young people with bipolar disorder are especially prone to rapid cycling or mixed episodes. Lithium may be less likely to be effective for people with these mood patterns, but anticonvulsants such as Depakote and Tegretol show promise in such cases. The medication options also include atypical antipsychotics, antidepressants, and anti-anxiety medications. In practice, it's often necessary for teens to take multiple medicines to manage all their symptoms.

Even after your teen starts to feel better, long-term medication is frequently needed to minimize the risk of future mood episodes. Changing or stopping the medication too soon may just lead to a recurrence.

One last, unusual thing about mood-stabilizing medications: Some teens may resist taking them even when they work very well. That's because, while some folks find the symptoms of mania disturbing, others find them exhilarating—at least, until the high starts to fade and they see the havoc their illness has caused. One mother, whose young adult son had just been released from the hospital the day before, wrote in an e-mail: "My son loves being manic (he feels like he is the king of the world), and the meds bring him down, so he hates them. Four out of his six hospitalizations happened because he went off his meds." It may help if you can find a doctor your teen really trusts and listens to. Hopefully, that trusted voice along with your own guidance will steer your teen toward making good choices as he or she gets older.

*"My son loves being manic (he feels like he is the king of the world), and the meds bring him down, so he hates them."*

### Why Is Psychotherapy a Valuable Adjunct to Medication?

Bipolar disorder is a multifaceted illness that calls for a multidimensional treatment approach. Along with medication, psychotherapy is an essential part of any comprehensive treatment plan. This may be particularly important for young people, since research shows that early psychological and social impairment lays the groundwork for continuing problems later in life. On the other hand, early, effective treatment may start adolescents down an altogether healthier life path.

The types of psychotherapy described under Treatment of Depression (pp. 73–76) in this chapter are generally applicable to bipolar disorder as well. The general issues involved in psychotherapy are discussed in detail there. The potential benefits for adolescents with bipolar disorder include:

- less denial about the seriousness of the disease
- better adherence to the medication plan
- increased ability to handle symptoms effectively
- improved functioning at home and school

For people with bipolar disorder, traditional psychotherapy may be combined with social rhythm therapy, which attempts to regularize their daily routines. It has been found that regular daily routines and sleep schedules may help people with bipolar disorder keep their moods on a more even keel.

As with depression, it's important that psychotherapy for bipolar disorder be provided by a therapist with training and experience in treating this illness. Since medication is used as well, the therapist should be willing to coordinate efforts with the prescribing doctor. The strong genetic component of bipolar disorder means that it's not uncommon for another family member living in the same household to have a mood disorder as well. In such cases, it's vital that everyone who needs treatment gets it, since a manic episode in one person may set off an emotional chain reaction among other members of the family.

In addition, the family as a whole may benefit from family therapy. Stress and conflict at home can play a role in triggering mood episodes. A teen's manic behavior, in turn, can quickly ratchet up the stress and strain for everyone else. It's little surprise, then, that several studies of people who have recently been hospitalized for bipolar disorder have found that those who returned home to a stressful environment were at increased risk for relapse. On the other hand, a calmer home makes life more pleasant for everyone while reducing the relapse risk for the teen with bipolar disorder.

*A calmer home makes life more pleasant for everyone . . .*

Family therapy can help your family work together as a unit toward this goal.

## What Other Treatments May Be Helpful?

Occasionally, someone in the grips of a manic episode doesn't respond adequately to the combination of medication and psychotherapy, even after several different medication regimens have been tried. If the symptoms are severe or if there is a concern about suicide, electroconvulsive therapy (ECT) offers another option. ECT involves the administration of a short series of carefully controlled electrical pulses to the brain, which produces a brief seizure. The procedure is described in detail in the Treatment of Depression section (pp. 82–84) of this chapter. Research has shown that ECT may be helpful for people with severe mania that doesn't improve with other treatments.

Some people with bipolar disorder notice that the depressive phase of their illness tends to follow a seasonal pattern, starting in fall or winter and subsiding in the spring. Such people may benefit from light therapy, in which they're treated throughout the dark winter months with daily exposure to very bright light from an artificial source. For a full description of light therapy, see the Treatment of Depression section (pp. 80–82) of this chapter. People with bipolar disorder need to approach this treatment carefully, however, because it may have the potential to trigger a switch from depression to mania. Although the special light boxes used in light therapy are sold without a prescription, they should only be utilized under the guidance of an experienced doctor or therapist.

## Handling a Suicidal Crisis

One of the most frightening prospects for any parent is the possibility of suicide. If your teen acts or talks in a way that leads you to believe that he or she might be feeling suicidal, get help immediately. Contact your child's doctor, a therapist, or a community mental health agency right away. To find a crisis center in your area, call the National Hopeline Network at 1-800-SUICIDE (784-2433). Or dial 911, if necessary. Don't try to handle the crisis alone.

Even if there are no overt signs of suicidal thoughts or feelings, you may still be concerned because of your teen's mood disorder. Don't be afraid to start a dialogue on the subject. Contrary to popular belief, talking about suicide won't put ideas in your child's head. Instead, it opens the door to frank discussion. If your teen does share some suicidal thoughts or plans, try to stay calm, but don't underreact. Stress that suicide is a permanent response to a temporary problem. Then outline steps the two of you can take together to get help and find a better alternative.

## Finding a Mental Health Professional

Few treatment decisions are more important than the choice of a treatment provider for your adolescent. In many cases, your teen may actually have two providers: a physician who prescribes and monitors medication therapy, and a therapist who provides psychotherapy. Ideally, these providers would each have substantial training and experience in adolescent mental health care. Unfortunately, the reality often falls far short of this ideal, especially for families who have limited resources or who live in rural areas. "There's no psychiatrist at all around here," says one mother. "We live up in the mountains, and the closest psychiatrist is an hour and a half away."

To understand the scope of the problem, consider the fact that there are only about 7,000 child and adolescent psychiatrists in the whole United States. Of course, psychiatrists who treat mainly adults often see some younger patients as well. In many cases, though, the medical management of adolescent depression or bipolar disorder is overseen by pediatricians and other primary care physicians. While such physicians can prescribe psychiatric medications, they don't have the extensive training of a specialist, and it's doubtful that most have the time to keep up with the latest advances in the diagnosis and treatment of mental disorders.

Unless your teen's symptoms are very mild, it's usually best to ask the primary care physician for a referral to a mental health specialist. If you're lucky enough to have several treatment providers from whom to choose, be sure to compare their training and experience specifically in the area of adolescent mood disorders. Other factors to consider include a provider's treatment approach, fees and payment policies, the type of insurance accepted, and office hours and location.

It's important that your adolescent feels comfortable with the treatment provider you ultimately select. But it's helpful if *you* and the provider can establish good rapport as well. As the mother of two sons with bipolar disorder explains: "One hallmark of a good provider is his willingness to work with the whole family and to include the parents in the plan of care. Remember: A critical component of a good outcome is a caring, educated family. I feel like my son's doctor and I have a true collaboration based on mutual respect."

*"I feel like my son's doctor and I have a true collaboration based on mutual respect."*

**Mental Health Professionals**

Several different kinds of professionals provide mental health services.

| Health care professional | May prescribe medication? | May provide psychotherapy? |
|---|---|---|
| Psychiatrists | Yes | Yes |
| Primary care physicians | Yes | No |
| Psychiatric nurses | Yes, with advanced training | Yes |
| Clinical psychologists | No* | Yes |
| Clinical social workers | No | Yes |
| Mental health counselors | No | Yes |
| Marriage and family therapists | No | Yes |

*New Mexico and Louisiana recently passed laws that grant prescribing privileges to clinical psychologists with advanced training. At this writing, the laws were still in the process of being implemented.

## Making Choices About Hospitalization

Most treatment for depression or bipolar disorder is provided on an outpatient basis. If your adolescent's symptoms become very severe, however, hospitalization may be recommended to keep your teen safe until the situation is less volatile. Inpatient care in a hospital setting may be helpful if your adolescent:

- poses a threat to himself or herself, or to others
- is behaving in a bizarre or destructive manner
- requires medication that must be closely monitored
- needs round-the-clock care to become stabilized
- has not improved in outpatient care

Today, inpatient hospitalization is generally used for short-term treatment to stabilize an adolescent's condition. Teens go home as quickly as possible, which minimizes the disruption to family life. Of course, this also reduces the cost for managed care plans, which may be loath to foot expensive hospital bills.

Whatever the reason, the average stay in psychiatric hospitals is now measured in days. Intermediate services can help a teen who is ready to leave the hospital but who still needs specialized care. For example, partial hospitalization programs provide intensive treatment during the day but allow the teen to go home at night.

The decision to hospitalize a child is a high-anxiety moment for most parents. For an adolescent in crisis, though, the 24-hour care and intensive support may be critical. Marcus and Jeanne say their 17-year-old daughter's recent hospitalization for mania marked a turning point for the better:

Kendra has been on medication for bipolar disorder since she was 11. After 6 years, her parents thought taking medication was such a deeply ingrained habit that they could safely let Kendra assume more responsibility for herself. "We thought, we're going to start prepping her for adulthood," says Jeanne. In late May, Kendra secretly stopped taking her medication, but it wasn't until early June that her parents realized something was terribly wrong.

"She was cutting herself, she was argumentative about everything, she got arrested for possession of marijuana. It was horrible," Jeanne recalls. Kendra began telling people she didn't want to go home because her parents abused her. One day, she called Social Services and reported the same thing. The next morning, she ran away. Finally, in desperation, her parents called for help, and Kendra was admitted to the child psychiatric unit of the local hospital.

"At the hospital, they forced her to go back on medication," says Marcus. "And they got her to open up." In group therapy, Kendra was able to share her feelings in a way she hadn't done before. As her mood became more stable, she was able to own up for the first time to the hurt she had caused herself and other people.

"It was heart-wrenching for all of us," says Jeanne. "But it was an eye-opening experience for Kendra." Jeanne credits hospitalization with helping her daughter come to better terms with herself, her illness, and the consequences of stopping medication.

*Jeanne credits hospitalization with helping her daughter come to better terms with herself, her illness, and the consequences of stopping medication.*

## What if Your Teen Doesn't Consent to Hospitalization?

Many parents are surprised to learn that their teenage child under age 18 may have certain rights to refuse treatment, including hospitalization. The nature of the rights and the age at which they begin vary from state to state. However, it's quite possible that you could find yourself in a situation where your teen's psychiatrist recommends hospitalization, and you agree, but your teen doesn't consent. In such cases, most states allow a physician to prescribe involuntary hospitalization for a short evaluation period, usually 3 days.

After that 3-day period is up, if the evaluation team believes that a longer hospitalization is needed, a court hearing is required to determine whether the teen can be forced to stay in the hospital. If involuntary admission is recommended, the court is able to issue an order for a specific period of time. In practice, though, it may be difficult to get such an order because of concerns about violating the teen's civil liberties.

This is a tricky situation, because most parents share the court's concern for their teen's rights. Nevertheless, a teenager who is immature and whose judgment may be impaired by illness often doesn't have the life experience or insight to make good treatment decisions. The hospital staff or an attorney may be able to advise you about your options in this situation, but it's a complex problem that may not have an easy solution.

## Finding Other Mental Health Services

Hospitalization is just one of many treatment options. These options lie on a continuum, with inpatient hospital care at one extreme and occasional outpatient visits to a therapist or physician at the other. In between, there are a number of other possibilities for accessing treatment and support services:

- Residential treatment centers—Facilities that provide round-the-clock supervision and care in a dorm-like group setting. The treatment is less specialized and intensive than in a hospital, but the length of stay is often considerably longer.
- Crisis residential treatment services—Temporary, 24-hour care in a nonhospital setting during a crisis; for example, if a teen becomes aggressive at home. The goal is to give an explosive situation time to cool off and to plan for what comes next in the teen's treatment.
- Partial hospitalization or day treatment—Services such as individual and group therapy, special education, vocational training, parent counseling, and therapeutic recreational activities that are provided for at least 4 hours per day. The adolescent gets intensive services during the day but is able to go home at night.
- Home-based services—Assistance provided in the adolescent's home; for example, help with implementing a behavior therapy plan or training for parents and teens on managing the illness. The goal is to improve family coping skills and avert the need for more expensive services, such as hospitalization.
- Respite care—Child care provided by trained parents or mental health aides for a short period of time. The goal is to give families a much-needed breather from the strain of caring for an ill teen.

To locate treatment and support services in your community, ask your teen's doctor or therapist for a referral. You might also try asking other parents, your teen's school counselor, your own doctor, a clergyperson, social service agencies, or the mental health division of your local health department.

## What Is a Systems of Care Approach?

For adolescents with severe mental illness, it's especially helpful if standard treatment can be combined with other support services. Ideally, such services should be part of what's known as a system of care—in other words, a network of mental health and social services that are organized to work together to provide care for a particular adolescent and his or her family. The idea is that, since mental illness touches every facet of a young person's life, optimal treatment may require many kinds of services from a variety of sources. These sources include not only traditional mental health facilities but also schools and social service organizations.

*. . . optimal treatment may require many kinds of services from a variety of sources.*

Within an ideal system, local public and private organizations team up to plan and implement an individualized set of services that are tailored to your adolescent's emotional, physical, educational, social, and family needs. Depending on the situation, your teen's team might include representatives that specialize in family advocacy, mental health, medicine, education, child welfare, juvenile justice, vocational counseling, substance abuse counseling, or recreational activities. A case manager serves as the team coordinator, keeping lines of communication open and tying together the entire bundle of services. Meanwhile, the team as a whole strives to build on your teen's strengths as well as address any problems. Of all the team members, none has a more important role to play than you and your adolescent. Both of you should be integral parts of team decision making about the care that is provided.

At least, that's the way things are supposed to work. In reality, such careful coordination of services is often the happy exception rather than the rule. Some families may have trouble getting special education services for a teen at school or finding community-based services for after-school hours. Other families may not have access to the home-based services that can help improve a teen's ability to function in the family and sometimes avert the need for hospitalization.

When such support services are available, however, they can be a valuable addition to psychotherapy and medication. Donna, for instance, is the mother of two sons who developed severe mental illness during their teens. "A TSS [therapeutic support staff person] would come out to the house and work on a behavior plan that had been set up by the behavior therapist. Since I had two sick kids—one with bipolar disorder, and the other with schizoaffective disorder—we had these services for years, and it really made a difference," Donna says. For suggestions on getting the full range of services your teen needs, see the next section of this chapter titled Navigating the Mental Health System and the section of Chapter 4 titled Working With the School (pp. 134–145).

## Falling Through the Cracks

A wide array of mental health services have been developed in recent decades. Yet the majority of adolescents with mental illness are still not receiving treatment of any kind. A recent telephone survey sponsored by the Annenberg Public Policy Center of the University of Pennsylvania sheds light on this situation. The survey, conducted between September and December 2003, included a national, representative sample of 506 primary care physicians. Only 46% of the doctors said they felt "very capable" of recognizing depression in their adolescent patients, and just 16% felt very capable of identifying bipolar disorder. In addition, only one in three doctors said they thought their community offered adequate treatment resources for adolescents with mental disorders, and more than half strongly believed that lack of insurance coverage hindered teenagers' ability to get the treatment they needed.

## Navigating the Mental Health System

Identifying appropriate services and choosing a qualified provider are steps in the right direction. Yet, for many parents, the biggest challenge still lies ahead: finding a way to foot the bill for these services. Some families lack any insurance coverage at all for mental health services, while others who do have insurance often find that the coverage is woefully inadequate. Nearly all private insurance plans impose some restrictions on mental health benefits, such as limiting the number of outpatient sessions or inpatient days that are covered. Some plans also require higher copayments and deductibles for mental health services. In addition, private insurance usually doesn't cover the full spectrum of community- and home-based services that teens with severe depression or bipolar disorder may urgently need in order to continue living at home.

*"I've spent tens of thousands of dollars for care that wasn't covered by insurance."*

"I've spent tens of thousands of dollars for care that wasn't covered by insurance," says the father of two teens with mood disorders. "But I know I'm one of the lucky ones, because I had the money to do it. I met a mother about a month ago who had lost her house and her car, because she used the money to take care of a child with bipolar disorder." It's the kind of family tragedy that is played out all too often.

### What Publicly Funded Services Are Available?

By far the biggest payer for community- and home-based services is Medicaid, a government program, paid for by a combination of federal and state funds, that provides health and mental health care to low-income individuals who meet eligibility criteria. Medicaid is supplemented by the State Child Health Insurance Program (SCHIP), which provides coverage for children whose families have a slightly higher income level. Some states put their SCHIP children into their regular Medicaid program, but others provide SCHIP children with private insurance, which is subject to the same limitations as other private insurance plans.

Unfortunately, since both Medicaid and SCHIP have financial eligibility requirements, many middle-class families don't qualify. These families find themselves in a classic double bind: They don't make enough money to pay for costly mental health services out of pocket, but they make too much to qualify for government programs. In some places, such families are advised to relinquish custody of their children to the state in order to gain access to the care they need. In other places, parents are told to call the police and turn their children over to the juvenile justice system in order to get needed services. It's a non-solution that subverts the true purpose of the child welfare and juvenile justice systems while forcing parents to make excruciating choices.

To help families who might otherwise be caught in this bind, federal law offers the states a couple of options. The best known is the TEFRA option, authorized by the Tax Equity and Financial Responsibility Act of 1982; it's also called the Katie Beckett option after the child whose situation originally inspired it. TEFRA allows states to cover community- and home-based services for children with disabilities who are living at home and need extensive care, regardless of family income. However, such flexibility comes at a price for the states. As of 2002, only 10 states had chosen to offer the TEFRA option to children with mental and emotional disorders. To find out more about Medicaid and related options in your state, check the phone book government pages, or visit the Centers for Medicare and Medicaid Services at www.cms.hhs.gov.

If gaining access to treatment for your teen sounds a bit hit or miss, it is. "We don't have a system of mental health care in the United States so much as lots of fractured pieces of a system," says Melissa Morton Lackman, an attorney who chairs the Legal Advocacy Council of the Child and Adolescent Bipolar Foundation (CABF). Parents who learn how to work the "system," such as it is, can sometimes get needed services. "But even if you're educated and resourceful, you have to know the right questions to ask," says Lackman. Parent and patient support groups, such as CABF and the Depression and Bipolar Support Alliance (DBSA), may be good starting points for learning the ropes.

Not surprisingly, many parents say that financial concerns are among the most stressful aspects of raising an adolescent with depression or bipolar disorder. Thousands of parents each year make the painful choice to give up custody of their children in order to get them the care they need. Others intentionally let their careers slide so that they can qualify for low-income programs. And still others with good jobs and above-average benefits nevertheless find themselves in an exhausting, never-ending struggle to make ends meet. As one mother, whose husband is a successful consulting engineer, says: "I think it's the financial commitment that overwhelms my husband. It doesn't matter how hard he works or how much money he makes. There's never enough. We haven't gone on a real vacation in four years. We don't have money to go out or fix up our house. Every penny goes to taking care of the kids, and it's still not enough."

*"Every penny goes to taking care of the kids, and it's still not enough."*

### What Is Mental Health Parity?

Mental health parity is a policy that attempts to stop the discrimination by insurance plans against mentally ill individuals that is so widespread today. The goal is to equalize the way that mental and physical illnesses are covered. The Mental Health Parity Act of 1996 was a tentative first step in that direction. This federal law applies only to employers with more than 50 workers. It states that, if an employer's group health plan includes any mental health coverage, the plan can't impose annual or lifetime dollar limits on mental health benefits that are lower than those for medical or surgical benefits. Yet the law falls short of guaranteeing true parity. For one thing, it doesn't require group health plans to include any mental health coverage at all. For another, it doesn't apply to group health plans sponsored by employers with 50 or fewer workers. It also doesn't ban health plans from using tactics to skirt the spirit of the law, such as imposing limits on the number of covered visits or requiring higher copayments for mental health services.

A number of states have also enacted their own mental health parity legislation. Like the federal law, however, most of these

---

### Startling Stats

- Approximate cost of a single outpatient therapy session: $100
- Average cost of inpatient care for youths who need psychiatric hospitalization: $7181 for bipolar disorder and $5288 for depression
- Approximate cost of 1 year at a residential treatment center: $250,000
- Percentage of private insurance plans that put restrictions on mental health benefits: 94% to 96%, depending on the type of plan
- Estimated annual number of U.S. children placed in the child welfare or juvenile justice systems solely to obtain mental health services: 12,700

state laws have significant gaps in the protections they offer. Several mental health advocacy groups are currently working to get more comprehensive legislation passed. If you're interested in learning more or getting involved in advocacy efforts, the National Alliance for the Mentally Ill and National Mental Health Association are good places to start.

### How Should You Choose a Managed Care Plan?

If your family does have mental health coverage through either private insurance or Medicaid, chances are good that you'll be dealing with a managed care organization. Managed care is a system for controlling health care costs. There are several different types of managed care plans, including:

- Health maintenance organization (HMO)—In this type of plan, you must use health care providers who work for the HMO. If services from an outside mental health care provider are needed, you usually must get a referral from your primary care doctor.
- Preferred provider organization (PPO)—In this type of plan, you may choose from a network of providers who have contracts with the PPO. You're less likely to need a referral from your primary care doctor to get access to a mental health care provider.
- Point of service (POS) plan—This type of plan is similar to a traditional HMO or PPO, except that you can also use providers outside the HMO organization or PPO network. You generally must pay a higher copayment or deductible for out-of-network care.

If you have a choice among several managed care plans, be sure to compare the benefit packages carefully. Watch out for clauses that exclude certain mental health diagnoses or services,

## Dos and Don'ts of Managed Care

*Do . . .*

- familiarize yourself with the provisions of your health plan.
- get to know your primary care provider as soon as possible.
- become actively involved in planning services for your teen.
- know in advance whom to call and where to go in an emergency.
- get any required preauthorization for nonemergency services.
- learn about the procedure for appealing a treatment denial.

*Don't . . .*

- give up too quickly; persistence often pays off in appeals.
- forget to provide positive feedback when things go smoothly.

or that impose a waiting period or deny coverage for preexisting conditions. Also, check for clauses that restrict covered services, such as caps on the number of outpatient visits allowed per year or exclusions of certain medications from the approved drug list. If you already have a favorite doctor or therapist, make sure he or she is in the provider network. Otherwise, look for a comprehensive network, including some providers located near your home. Finally, consider the copayments and deductibles you'll have to pay. And try to get a feel for the administrative hassles you'll face once you actually try to access care.

### How Can You Influence Managed Care Decisions?

One of the main cost-cutting tools used by managed care plans is utilization review, a formal review of health care services to determine whether payment for them should be authorized or denied. In making this determination, the managed care company considers two factors: whether the services are covered under your health insurance plan and whether the services meet the standard for "medical necessity." To satisfy this standard, a health care service must be deemed medically appropriate and necessary to meet an individual's health care needs. Most treatment denials are based on the medical necessity provision. This is a situation in which your health insurance plan covers the services a doctor or therapist recommends, but the managed care company decides not to pay for them anyway because they aren't deemed medically necessary. Needless to say, this can be an extremely frustrating situation.

For example, Lisa says that her health plan initially authorized an emergency hospitalization for her son at the closest available facility, even though it wasn't in the plan's care network. The next morning, however, "they wanted us to move him, despite the fact that he was in a very fragile state. He was catatonic. I fought with the insurance company, and I was finally told he could stay." A few weeks later, though, Lisa was surprised to receive a sizable bill. Despite what the representative had told her on the phone, the health plan had denied coverage for part of her son's hospitalization, claiming it wasn't medically necessary for him to remain in that particular facility.

Fortunately, managed care companies that use a utilization review process are also required to offer an appeals process for services that are denied. If you file an appeal, enlist the help of the health care provider who originally recommended the treatment. When you're seeking preapproval for emergency services, an expedited appeals process should be available. But if it's after the fact or the situation isn't an emergency, getting a decision may take some time. In Lisa's case, it took more than three months, but she finally succeeded in getting her health plan to cover her son's entire hospital stay.

*If you file an appeal, enlist the help of the health care provider who originally recommended the treatment.*

If your first appeal is denied, request written notification of the reasons. This notice should also explain what information would be needed for the treatment to be approved. You can always appeal again. Most managed care companies have three or four levels of appeal, and each involves a different set of people. Eventually, you may be able to make your case successfully.

If you encounter problems at any point in the appeals process, there are sources of outside help. For insurance that is provided by an employer, the human resources department may be able to assist you. For Medicaid issues, your state may have an ombudsman, a person whose job it is to investigate and try to resolve consumer complaints. Local mental health organizations may also be able to provide helpful advice or recommend useful resources. If all your appeals have been exhausted, the managed care company and your provider should agree upon an acceptable alternative to the treatment that was originally requested.

Throughout this whole process, you can play an active role in advocating for your child's treatment needs. Although it may seem daunting at first, many parents learn to become very effective in this role. Following are some parting thoughts from parents who started out just as lost and confused as you may be feeling right now, but who eventually found their way through the managed care maze:

"Almost every hospitalization, I've had to fight with the insurance companies, but ultimately I won. I document *everything*, and I just don't give up. You have to be relentless."

"At one point, I had something like 60 days of hospitalization available to my daughter and only $500 in therapy. I called the insurance company and convinced them to give us more therapy dollars as a tradeoff for some of the hospitalization days."

"I document everything, and I just don't give up. You have to be relentless."

"A lot of people would be told it's not covered and let it go at that. Well, let me tell you something: I've had to push, but I've been successful 100% of the time up to this point. Right now, I'm in a battle with the insurance company about one of the meds our psychiatrist prescribed that they don't want to cover. That's when I get busy. I go out and research it. Sometimes, I actually write the letters that my doctor signs. You'd be surprised what they'll cover if you really push."

## Chapter Four

# Living Daily Life: Helping Your Teen at Home and School

G etting the best possible treatment for your adolescent with depression or bipolar disorder is your top priority. After that hurdle has been crossed, however, you may soon realize that there are still many challenges left to overcome. Depression and bipolar disorder affect every aspect of your teen's functioning at home and school. As a parent, there are steps you can take to help things go more smoothly in these key areas of daily life. By reducing stress this way, you may also help speed your teen's recovery and reduce the chances of a relapse or recurrence.

Adolescence is by definition a time of transition from childhood to adulthood. It's a period when children naturally start to pull away from their parents and begin to forge independent lives and identities. For both you and your teen, this transition involves major changes in roles and expectations. At times, the changes can be exhilarating, and at other times, they can be rather frightening. For parents of a teen with depression and bipolar disorder, the anxiety may be magnified. However, the push-pull of autonomy versus dependence is something that all parents of adolescents go through. It's a natural phase in the evolution of your role as a parent.

While your relationship with your teen will inevitably change, that doesn't mean it becomes any less significant. In fact, your teen may need the security of your steadfast love and support more than ever now. The way you communicate with your adolescent and structure your family life can have a major impact on how your teen functions at home— which, in turn, can influence how your teen functions in other situations. The time and energy you devote to your other children, your significant other, and yourself can help keep the teen's issues in perspective—a good thing for all of you. And the way you address school issues and advocate for your teenager's educational needs can have a decisive impact on his or her success in school.

*. . . your teen may need the security of your steadfast love and support more than ever*

All the while, you'll be slowly but surely working toward one of the most difficult but ultimately gratifying tasks for any parent: letting go. As the parent of an adolescent with depression or bipolar disorder, you may have to take things a bit more gradually than other parents, but the ultimate goal of helping your child move toward a healthy, productive, independent life as a young adult is still the same. Miriam is one mother who has helped her daughter make the transition successfully:

> Allie had been diagnosed with bipolar disorder at age 7, and her teenage years were often bumpy. "She was being picked on by some of the other kids, and her reaction to that was to get loud. She was the one who was always punished," Miriam remembers. "She also seemed to develop a pattern starting in middle school of making herself seem even more different from the other kids. For example, the first two years of high school, she got very interested in the pagan earth religions thing, and she would be sure to tell the most conservative Christian kids in her school about it." As the teasing from other students intensified, so did Allie's anger. By tenth grade, the situation had become so volatile that Miriam decided to homeschool her daughter.

Away from the "hot" environment at school, Allie began to thrive. Her angry outbursts subsided, and her engagement in positive activities, such as private voice lessons, improved. Allie and her mother found creative ways to meet her academic requirements, even while her mother continued to work as a public relations executive. Despite the nontraditional education, Allie did very well on her SATs and was easily able to get into a good college.

Getting accepted by a college was only half the battle, however. "Allie was doing much better, but she still had emotional meltdowns," says her mother. "One of the parameters I set for her was that her college couldn't be more than an hour or two from home." Allie settled upon a small liberal arts university about an hour away. For two years, she did well in her studies, despite the occasional "meltdown," while she nurtured a strong literary flare. Then the budding writer, with her mother's blessing, did what so many writers before have done: headed for New York City. Allie is now in her senior year at a university there, and her mother proudly notes that "she's doing poetry readings in some of the premier venues and selling her little poetry books."

How did they get from violent blowups to poetry readings? Miriam says, "The most important thing is to really think it through and break down all the skills that your child needs to have. And try to set up situations in which she's independent, but you're right there nearby, so that if she falls, you can be there to pick her up before anything too bad happens." Over time, you'll reach the point where you can safely stand farther and farther away, until you finally let go altogether.

> "The most important thing is to really think it through and break down all the skills that your child needs to have."

## Communicating With Your Teen

Before your child reaches the promised land of adulthood, however, you'll need to guide him or her down the sometimes-rocky path of adolescence. Difficulties with communication are among the first obstacles you're likely to meet. It's not uncommon for teens to stop talking to their parents for any number of reasons. For example, they may be embarrassed about their new feelings and desires, or they may fear that they will be lectured or ridiculed if they share their beliefs. Depression may just exaggerate this tendency to withdraw, while mania may lead to the opposite extreme of uncontrollable volubility. Neither is very conducive to meaningful conversation. As one parent put it, "My daughter would go from not talking at all for days or weeks to screaming for hours on end."

Getting treatment for the mood episode is the first step toward reestablishing communication. Psychotherapy often helps develop communication skills directly, while medication may reduce related symptoms and help foster participation in psychotherapy. Once your adolescent's mood is more stable, it will be easier to start a real dialogue. Even if your teen acts uninterested at first, bear in mind that most young people really want to feel a close connection with their parents. Your teen may just need a signal that you want that, too, especially if there has been considerable tension in your relationship.

To start the ball rolling, ask about your adolescent's day, and talk about your own. At home, put limits on television and computer time. In the car, switch off the cell phone and turn down the music. Then spend more time relating to one another instead. If your teen is reluctant to talk at first, make it clear that you just want to build mutual understanding, not find fault. Rather than forcing a conversation, nudge your teen in that direction by learning about his or her personal interests.

Once your adolescent starts to open up, be an attentive listener. You don't have to agree with everything your teen says, but be open-minded. If your teen shares an idea that seems silly or immature, give it a serious hearing nonetheless. If your teen shares a mistake, make it clear that you accept him or her even if you reject the behavior. Then try to help your teen find the lesson in the experience.

When the time seems right, don't be afraid to bring up sensitive topics, such as substance abuse, sexual activity, or thoughts of self-injury or suicide. In fact, these may be some of the issues your adolescent needs to talk about the most. It's best to broach these topics *before* a crisis occurs rather than waiting until you're already faced with an emergency. And don't hesitate to open a frank discussion about your teen's mental illness. By talking about depression or bipolar disorder as an illness that can be treated and managed like any other, you help instill a realistic yet hopeful attitude in your teen.

> It's best to broach these topics before a crisis occurs . . .

Unfortunately, some of your teen's peers may not be quite so enlightened. The pressure to conform to peer expectations can be intense at this age, and some teenagers may be quite cruel to those who are perceived as being different from the norm. Mental illness is one difference that sets your teen apart. When you add other factors—anything from belonging to a racial, ethnic, or religious minority group, to being very short or overweight, to having a learning disorder or physical disability— the harassment may become even more vicious or relentless. If you suspect that your teen might be the target of teasing or bullying, bring up the subject. Let your adolescent know that it isn't his or her fault, and reassure your teen that it doesn't have to be faced alone. Then start a discussion about ways of handling the situation.

Ultimately, you want your adolescent to know that you're available to discuss *anything* that may be troubling him or her, whatever the problem might be. Sometimes, your teen may be seeking advice on a solution. Other times, your teen may simply want a

## Bully-Busting Tips

"Other kids view him as quirky and not fitting in, so he's had a rough time. He got beat up one year by a group of kids at school." It's a common lament among parents of adolescents with depression or bipolar disorder. Here are some suggestions for helping your teen cope with bullying:

- Build your teen's self-confidence, which is a deterrent to bullies.

- Encourage your teen to stay in a group, since bullies like to target loners.

- Tell your teen to try not to show fear or anxiety, since bullies feed off these kinds of emotional reactions. Instead, your teen might simply walk away or use humor to defuse the situation.

- Teach your teen to respond with assertiveness, not aggressiveness. Simply saying "stop that!" in a confident voice may be helpful, but fighting back only throws more fuel on the fire.

- Urge your teen to report the bullying immediately to a trusted adult. If the bullying is occurring at school, it's also appropriate for you to let the principal know about the problem.

- Refer your teen to the Stop Bullying Now! website (www.stopbullyingnow.hrsa.gov), sponsored by the U.S. Department of Health and Human Services.

- Talk about the value of individual differences. One mother of two teenagers with bipolar disorder handled the subject this way: "Yes, you're different, but everybody's different. Just because you see life differently and learn differently doesn't mean you're wrong."

sounding board for bouncing off his or her own ideas. In either case, you're fulfilling a vital need for adult guidance and parental support. The alternative is to let your child learn about life strictly from friends and the media—poor substitutes for the wisdom, experience, and values a parent can impart.

## How Should You Address Your Teen's Illness?

As a parent, your natural instinct is to protect your child. When it comes to the realities of depression or bipolar disorder, however, you may do more harm than good by trying to shield your adolescent from the whole truth. Your teen is already well aware that something is amiss. Kept in the dark, he or she may conclude that the situation is much bleaker than it really is. The truth, by comparison, is actually rather reassuring. Yes, your teen has an illness. It's a fact of his or her life that needs to be accepted. But it's also a very treatable condition—not an insurmountable barrier to health or happiness.

*Yes, your teen has an illness. . . . But it's also a very treatable condition.*

When your adolescent shares concerns about the disease, try to stifle the impulse to respond with false comfort. If you say things are fine when they emphatically are not, your teen may become demoralized by the thought that this is as good as it gets. Or your teen may question how you could ever understand *anything* when you're so clearly out of touch with what he or she is thinking, feeling, and experiencing. Instead, acknowledge that your adolescent is indeed having a tough time right now, but also let your teen know that this difficult period won't last forever.

Once your adolescent begins to confide in you, be sensitive about how you use this information. There will be times when you need to reach out to others for advice or support, and there are also people who have a legitimate reason to know what's going on in your teen's life. However, your teen also needs to feel that you can be trusted to respect his or her privacy. As with everything else, it's best to talk about this honestly. If your teen strongly prefers that you not discuss his or her problems with a certain person—for example, a family friend, a favorite aunt, or another sibling—ask yourself whether this other party really needs to be informed.

---

### What's in a Name?

When talking to your adolescent and those closest to your family—other family members, close friends, and teachers, for instance—it makes sense to use precise medical terms for describing your teen's mood disorder. When talking to casual acquaintances or total strangers, however, you may have neither the time nor the inclination to explain what "depression" or "bipolar disorder" really means. To avoid misunderstanding in such cases, you may want to go with a more neutral-sounding name for your teen's illness. One parent says that, when her teen flies into a rage in public, onlookers often assume that the child is being abused and try to intervene. A curt explanation that the teen has a "neurological disorder" usually allays these well-meaning strangers' concerns.

---

## Managing Your Home Life

Another crucial way you can help your adolescent is by providing a home life that is conducive to getting better. Stability and structure are the name of the game. The more erratic and unpredictable your teen's behavior, the more everyone in the family benefits from a routine that seems comfortably calm and predictable. While a little variety may add spice to life, too much just creates chaos and confusion.

Unfortunately, it's all too easy for family life to become hijacked by the ups and downs of your teen's moods. In this kind of volatile environment, behavior can quickly spiral out of control, as the mother of a 15-year-old with bipolar disorder discovered: "My son would fly into rages and start rattling off profanities at my husband and myself. We tried to shield his little sister from it as much as possible, because she didn't need to hear that. But it became a daily battleground. You couldn't make any rules, because he would just go off the deep end every time. At one point, it got so bad that my husband was afraid to go to work, because he didn't know what my son was going to do. We felt like we were being held hostage in our own home."

*"We felt like we were being held hostage in our own home."*

When a situation reaches this point, family therapy combined with treatment for your adolescent may be needed to get things back on track as quickly as possible. The therapist should be able to suggest specific strategies for dealing with problems such as rages and defiance. As a general rule, however, your teen may not be capable of cooperating with even the best-laid behavior plan until after treatment has gotten his or her mood symptoms at least partially under control.

### How Can You Provide Consistent Parenting?

Whether you're implementing a prescribed behavior plan or just doing everyday parenting, try to be consistent in how you respond to your teen. Inconsistency only leads to confusion and breeds inappropriate behavior. Within the limits of your teen's behavioral capabilities at the time, set clear rules with well-defined consequences. Make sure the rules are appropriate to your child's age and maturity level. Then follow through on enforcing the rules just as you said you would.

Consistency needs to carry over not only from one day to the next but also from one adult to another. Make sure you, your partner, and the therapist are all on the same page. If applicable, try to enlist the support of noncustodial parents, grandparents, teachers, or other key adults in your teen's life as well.

Otherwise, you may inadvertently teach your teen to behave in a way that is quite different from what you intended. Sharlene learned this lesson the hard way:

"I parent one way; my husband parents another. He's the one who makes the rules and sticks with them. I'm the one who's around the kids more, and they wear me down, so I give in. I think sometimes my husband is too hard on the kids. He thinks I'm too lenient."

Sharlene says this difference in parenting style created some discipline problems with all three of her children. However, the problems were amplified in the two with mood disorders. "I thought I was being kinder to them, but what they really needed was consistency," she says, looking back. "They got mixed signals, so they learned to disrespect one parent—and that parent was me."

For Sharlene and her husband, family counseling helped them resolve their differences and present a more unified front to the children. "The counselor's office was neutral ground," Sharlene says. "My husband and I would go in there, and the counselor would say, 'Okay, this is how you need to parent.' Neither one of us was right or wrong. It was just about learning how to discipline so it worked best for the kids."

> "The counselor's office was neutral ground."

### How Should You Handle Out-of-Control Behavior?

Some adolescents with depression or bipolar disorder may become very hostile, aggressive, or defiant. Others may lie, steal, stay out all night, run away from home, abuse drugs, or otherwise get into serious trouble. Such behavior may be a symptom of the mood disorder itself or of an associated condition, such as conduct disorder, oppositional defiant disorder, or substance abuse. Whatever label you put on the behavior, however, it's a major problem for parents who are trying to maintain a safe, orderly home for everyone in the family.

Parents of teens who are prone to this kind of behavior often report feeling as if they're walking on eggshells, because they never know what will set off the next crisis. This isn't a healthy environment for anyone, least of all your teen, who desperately needs to regain some sense of stability and control. Your family therapist or your teen's doctor should be able to provide suggestions for coping with this type of disruptive behavior. Ideally, you should have a contingency plan in place before a serious problem arises, so that you feel confident about your ability to handle whatever might come your way.

Don't panic if the unexpected does occur, however. Your anxiety will just fan the flames of your teen's emotions. Instead, look for ways to cool off the situation, such as stating firmly but calmly what you want your teen to do or walking away for a few minutes. Now is not the time for deep conversation, however. A teenager in the grips of an emotional outburst is in no frame of mind to think clearly or talk rationally.

During an outburst, your adolescent may say some very mean or hurtful things. Afterward, try to forget them as soon as possible. "Don't take it personally," advises one parent. "Realize that it's not really your kid talking; it's the illness. And try to understand that your child's behavior has nothing to do with you or the way you raised them. The illness can really bring out behaviors that you wouldn't normally see in that child."

### Defusing an Explosive Situation

If you're unable to get your adolescent's behavior under control in a reasonable amount of time, call for help. Sometimes, your spouse or another adult close to the teen may be able to defuse the situation. In addition, if your teenager appears to be a threat to anyone's safety, including his or her own, call your teen's doctor, a therapist, or a community mental health agency right away. If the danger seems imminent, take your teen to the emergency room, or call 911, if necessary.

## Parenting With a Partner

There's no doubt about it: Coping with the physical, emotional, and financial demands of raising a mentally ill adolescent can put a heavy strain on any marriage. Some don't survive, but other couples find that the challenge actually brings them closer and gives them a sense of shared purpose. How do they do it? Here are suggestions from some couples who have survived and thrived:

*"The children see that we're a partnership, and . . . that helps their behavior."*

- Make your marriage a priority. "Even though we have these children with problems, I think we put each other first. The children see that we're a partnership, and a lot of times that helps their behavior. They know they won't be able to play one parent against the other."

- Schedule regular time alone. "Spend some time with just each other. Going out can be really hard, because often you can't leave the kids alone, and grandma may not be able to handle them. But you still need to find a way, even if it's just to grab a cup of coffee together."

- Talk about your differences. "I tend to jump on things as soon as they happen, and my husband tends to minimize things. The psychiatrist said we have different realities, and until we find some way to bring our realities together, we're going to have trouble getting along."

- Consider marriage counseling. "We're starting marriage counseling in a week. I think for many years we just ignored our issues. We want to make sure our marriage doesn't slip through the cracks as our kids get older. You can create a lot of damage if you aren't careful."

## What if You're a Single Parent?

Parenting an adolescent with depression or bipolar disorder is challenging enough if you have a partner to help. For single parents, the challenges are even greater. Just because you aren't part of a couple doesn't mean you have to go it alone, however. Extended family and close friends can provide much-needed emotional support and practical help.

> "You need a support network," says Sara, who raised four children with mood disorders by herself for several years. "My family lives up in Canada, so family was out for me. But I have a lot of very good friends. Some of them would come over and sit with the kids from time to time—even for just a few hours once a month. That let me get out once in a while, and it really made a big difference."
>
> Over time, Sara gradually began dating again. "Once I started to get semi-serious with a guy, I would lay it on the line about the kids," she says. "It's not something you can hide. And I've had men walk away from the situation and say this was something they just couldn't deal with." Eventually, though, she met a man who stuck around. "He got used to the idea, and he became educated about it."
>
> Two years ago, Sara and the new man in her life got married. Since then, their focus has been on building a strong foundation for raising a family and learning to work together as a parenting team. "It hasn't been easy," says Sara. But she thinks that open communication and a strong commitment to each other are the keys.

## Dealing With Sibling Issues

When one family member has depression or bipolar disorder, it affects not only that person but everyone else in the household as well. Siblings may bear the brunt of a brother's or sister's angry outbursts, or they may mourn the loss of the close connection they once shared. Others simply get lost in all the commotion as parents struggle to cope with one crisis after another.

Younger siblings may learn by imitation that disruptive behaviors are a quick way to regain some of that lost attention. Older ones may drift away from the family, turning to other sources in an effort to get their emotional needs met. Some of these sources—such as sports teams or school clubs—may be healthy, but the draw of unhealthy choices—such as sex, drugs, or gangs—can be powerful.

Few parents set out to neglect any of their children. However, when you're feeling overburdened and exhausted, it's only natural to take the path of least resistance. Unfortunately, if you allow yourself to simply be swept along by events, you'll tend to be pulled toward the child with the problem and away from those who aren't as obviously demanding. It may take a conscious effort on your part to notice this tendency and work to correct it. Try to set aside some one-on-one time every day with each child. While this may seem like just one more task to squeeze into an already hectic schedule, it may actually save you time in the long run by cutting down on negative copycat behavior. At the very least, it will go a long way toward preserving the special bond you have with each of your children.

*Try to set aside some one-on-one time every day with each child.*

Another common problem is resentment caused by different rules for different children. One mother says that, when her 14-year-old daughter was at the low point of a depressive episode, "I didn't make her do chores, because she couldn't have done them. The younger one [a 13-year-old daughter] didn't like that and was pretty vocal about it." In this situation, it may help to have a frank talk with the unhappy sibling. Explain that you're not showing favoritism. You're actually treating each child exactly the same, by individualizing the rules for each based on his or her personal capabilities. It may help to point out that illness isn't the only reason why there might need to be different expectations for different children in the same family. For example, younger children aren't expected to do the same chores as older ones, but they're still expected to do tasks that are appropriate for their age and ability level.

Some siblings feel acutely embarrassed by the behavior of an ill brother or sister. That was the case for one family in which a teenage brother and sister went to the same high school. The girl, who had bipolar disorder, became very unruly during manic episodes. "There were times when they had to restrain her at school," their mother recalls, "and the other kids would be saying, 'Look at your crazy sister.'" On the one hand, she says, her son felt embarrassed. On the other, he felt protectiveness on behalf of his sister, with whom he had been very close when they were growing up. Such mixed feelings are quite common among family members. It may help you and your children alike to talk about them honestly when they occur.

## Taking Care of Yourself

Raising a teenager isn't easy. Raising a teenager with depression or bipolar disorder means doing all the stuff other parents do while also juggling doctor's appointments, therapist visits, medication schedules, insurance claims, school concerns, and a host of special behavioral issues. It's little wonder that some parents become overwhelmed by all the demands on their time and energy. When you start to feel this way, it's time to step back and take a hard look at your lifestyle.

Odds are, you'll find that you've become so consumed by taking care of everyone else that you forgot to take care of yourself.

*"My whole mission in life was just to get this kid stabilized."* One mother recalls that, for the first 6 months after her teenage son entered a manic phase, "I didn't even put in my contacts; I just wore my glasses. I didn't put on makeup. I didn't eat regularly. My whole mission in life was just to get this kid stabilized."

The irony is that, by neglecting your own needs, you're apt to become so exhausted and stressed that you're unable to be much use to anyone. To be at your best for your family, you need to be physically rested and mentally refreshed. When you think about it this way, taking 30 minutes to go for a walk, read a good book, visit with friends, or just sit quietly and meditate may be the most unselfish thing you could possibly do. Being a caregiver is more like running a marathon than a sprint, and you need to be healthy yourself if you plan to go the distance.

Another mother who has been coping with her son's bipolar disorder for several years now recalls that she was once one of the "martyr moms" as well. "Not anymore," she says. "I go to the gym and do Pilates—that's a sacrosanct hour. I have friends who I make the time to see. I get pedicures. You just have to find some time for yourself, even if it's only for an hour a week at first."

### Are You to Blame for Your Teen's Mood Disorder?

Parents often add to their own stress by blaming themselves for an adolescent's depression or bipolar disorder. Education may be the best antidote to this kind of misplaced guilt. Both depression and bipolar disorder are biological illnesses associated with changes in brain development, neurochemistry, and function. While environmental factors, including parenting, may influence the onset, severity, and recurrence of symptoms, other factors also affect the course of these diseases. It's not only inaccurate but also counterproductive to saddle yourself with the burden of needless self-blame.

Be alert for a related pitfall as well: It's all too easy to take knowledge about the biological basis of mood disorders and twist it around into finger-pointing of another kind. People may start blaming one side of the family or the other for passing on the depression or bipolar gene. "My ex-husband gave my children the gene. They never had a chance," says one mother. The truth is more complicated than that, however. Multiple genes are probably involved in mood disorders, and genetics is just one of the many contributors underlying these diseases.

It's certainly valid and maybe even useful to trace the genetic link between your adolescent and other relatives with mood disorders. However, the emphasis should always be on learning more about the illness and perhaps helping your teen appreciate the affinity he or she shares with other relatives who serve as positive role models. When the focus turns to placing blame, it becomes destructive. If that happens, you need to refocus on looking forward, rather than back.

### What if You Have a Mood Disorder, Too?

Because of the genetic component of mood disorders, it's not uncommon for a parent and child both to be affected. If that's your situation, it's important to seek treatment not only for your adolescent, but also for yourself. Families in which a parent has untreated mental illness tend to be characterized by less emotional support and more interpersonal conflict. These factors, in turn, may contribute to mood episodes and poor treatment adherence in children with depression or bipolar disorder.

By getting treatment and learning to manage your own symptoms, you make yourself more available to your adolescent—mentally, physically, and emotionally. You also model the good

## Dos and Don'ts of Work/Life Balance

*Do . . .*

- ask about insurance coverage for mental health care when considering a new job.
- enlist the help of human resources if you have problems with an insurance claim.
- try to negotiate flexible work hours to allow for potential family emergencies.
- carefully weigh whether to disclose your teen's condition to your employer.
- use your company's employee assistance program (EAP), if one is provided, as another source of mental health services for yourself and your family.
- know your rights under the Family and Medical Leave Act, which states that covered employers must grant eligible employees up to 12 work weeks of unpaid leave during any 12-month period to care for an immediate family member with a serious health condition. For details, visit the U.S. Department of Labor's Employment Standards Administration website at www.dol.gov/esa.

*Don't . . .*

- be afraid to explore creative options, such as job sharing or self-employment.
- let your job skills get rusty if you take a temporary break from your career; consider continuing ed classes or volunteer work to keep yourself marketable.

self-care habits you want your teen to learn. Interestingly, some parents who have neglected their own treatment over the years find that having an ill child motivates them to finally get the care they need. One mother, who was not formally diagnosed with bipolar disorder until her son was, says, "He's lucky, because he got help early. I don't want him to have to go through what I did as a teenager."

## Helping to Prevent a Recurrence of Your Teen's Illness

Even after your adolescent's condition has stabilized, there is still the possibility of a relapse or recurrence. You can play a central role in helping prevent future episodes by maintaining the health-promoting habits that were so important during your teen's healing process. Clear communication, a stable home life, a consistent parenting style, appropriate discipline, strong family bonds, positive role models, and good adherence to the maintenance treatment plan are all key ingredients in long-term success.

Throughout your teen's illness, try to become aware of his or her typical mood symptoms. That way, you can recognize the danger signs of an impending episode and get help at an early stage, before the symptoms have become too severe. You can help your adolescent learn to notice the warning flags as well.

### Been There, Done That

Do you ever feel as if no one really knows what you're going through? The authors of these books know, because they've been through it themselves as parents of children with depression or bipolar disorder. The books are testaments to the authors' steadfast determination to help their children and the hard-won insights they've gained along the way. The pages are filled with advice, inspiration, and a quiet courage you may find comfortingly familiar.

Lederman, Judith, and Candida Fink. *The Ups and Downs of Raising a Bipolar Child: A Survival Guide for Parents.* New York: Fireside, 2003.

Raeburn, Paul. *Acquainted With the Night: A Parent's Quest to Understand Depression and Bipolar Disorder in His Children.* New York: Broadway Books, 2004.

Steel, Danielle. *His Bright Light.* New York: Delacorte Press, 1998. (This is a loving memoir by the best-selling novelist, but be forewarned that the story of her son's life ends tragically in suicide.)

One mother, who is also a psychotherapist in her professional life, advises, "Become the one person your teen trusts to provide feedback about how she's acting. If you say, 'You're acting like you're depressed,' she needs to trust that feedback and match it up to her feelings and behaviors at the time." Eventually, this will help your teen learn to take prompt action and deal with mood symptoms as soon as they arise.

But while a little vigilance is a good thing, don't overdo it. Teenagers generally don't appreciate being smothered with parental attention. As another parent says, "What's important is not to hover over them, but to be available and aware of what's going on in their lives."

## Working With the School

Your adolescent spends more time at school than anywhere else but home. For teens, school is a place not only to learn about academic matters but also to connect with friends and get involved in extracurricular activities. Those who are successful in this setting acquire the cognitive and social skills they'll need later for college, work, and adult relationships. Unfortunately, teens with mood disorders are at high risk for poor attendance, academic underachievement, school failure, and dropping out. In the midst of an episode, they can find it very difficult to pay attention, think clearly, solve problems, recall information, sit still, and follow classroom rules.

*Once stabilized, it's quite possible for these teens to thrive in school*

Once stabilized, it's quite possible for these teens to thrive in school, but they may still need a little extra assistance from parents and teachers. Among other things, certain medications may cause side effects that detract from learning. These effects include drowsiness, fatigue, lack of mental alertness, memory problems, slurred speech, poor coordination, or physical discomforts, such as nausea or excessive thirst.

When confronted with a teen who has special needs, some teachers and administrators are quite adaptable and eager to help. Others, however, are inflexible and unsympathetic, based on ignorance or prejudice about mental disorders. Your challenge as a parent is to build an effective partnership with the school. Your goal is to support the positive teachers, educate the uninformed ones, and avoid the few who are unable to understand what your teen is experiencing.

To help your teen make the most of public school, you need to become aware of the educational opportunities that are available to students with disabilities, including those with mental illnesses. "The school system is the equal opportunity mental health provider, because if your child meets the eligibility requirements for IDEA [the Individuals with Disabilities Education Act], your income doesn't matter," says Tammy Seltzer, a senior staff attorney at the Bazelon Center for Mental Health Law. The schools are charged with providing a free and appropriate public education to all. For families whose income disqualifies them from Medicaid, the schools may be the best source of publicly funded services.

## How Can You Work Together With Your Teen's Teachers?

Teachers are your most important allies at school. They're the ones who spend an hour or more per day, five days a week, with your teen. And they're the ones who control the learning environment, for better or worse. When children are in elementary school, it's easy to get to know their teachers and perhaps volunteer at the school or help chaperone a field trip, if your schedule permits. As students get older, however, they may have a different teacher for each subject. Your teenage children may also seem considerably less enthusiastic about running into you in the hall at school.

Don't let this discourage you, however. No matter how they act, "kids of all ages really want their parents involved," says Donna Gilcher, a former teacher and school administrator who now directs educational programs for the Child and Adolescent Bipolar Foundation (CABF). Just be sensitive to your child's growing need for independence, especially in front of his or her friends. Says Gilcher, "In elementary school, it's okay to bring lunch up to your child and say, 'Honey, you forgot your lunch.' In middle school, you drop the lunch off in the office."

Make the extra effort to get acquainted with all your teen's teachers. "At the open house at the beginning of the year, I go up to the teachers and shake their hand," says one mother. "I look them right in the eye, and I hold their hand so they remember my face. I say, 'Hi, I'm Roberta Smith. I'm Jake's mom.' And then I say, 'Listen, if you have any problems, can you call me right away? Because we can chat about these things.' I make myself very approachable, and they call me."

*"I go up to the teachers and shake their hand"*

After the initial meeting, stay in touch throughout the year. If a problem develops, give the teacher the benefit of the doubt. Most teachers really want to do a good job for every student. Like parents, however, they may sometimes find it difficult to deal with a student whose behavior and learning ability are affected by a mood disorder or medication side effects. Approach the teacher with an attitude that says "we're all in this together," and you're much more likely to get a positive response. On the other hand, if you start out with an accusatory tone, the teacher's defenses will go up, and you're more likely to end up in an antagonistic posture.

Don't forget to also let the teacher know when things are going *right*. A occasional thank you note or small token of appreciation can help cement a strong alliance. You can also establish yourself as an asset to the school by participating in fund-raising efforts or volunteering in the office. Educators are only human; they respond to encouragement and support like anyone else. The more you can do to a build a positive working relationship with school personnel, the more effective you'll be when it comes time to request services for your student.

Occasionally, you may run across a teacher who remains unresponsive to your teen's needs, no matter what your approach. In such cases, it's perfectly appropriate to go to the principal with a complaint. Once again, though, try to avoid sounding accusatory when you state the problem. Instead, approach the principal with the attitude that this is a problem you can team up to solve together. That may be all it takes to enlist the teacher's cooperation. If all else fails, though, request a different placement for your student. Your teen has enough challenges in school without also having to cope with a teacher who is unwilling or unable to adapt to individual needs.

*Your teen has enough challenges in school without also having to cope with a teacher who is unwilling or unable to adapt to individual needs.*

## What Laws Cover Services for Students With Disabilities?

In the United States, there are two main laws that cover public school services for students with disabilities: IDEA and Section

504 of the Rehabilitation Act of 1973. IDEA is a federal law that applies to students who have a disability that impacts their ability to benefit from general educational services. In order to qualify for special services under IDEA, students must meet specific criteria within one of 13 categories of disability. The most obvious category for a teen with depression or bipolar disorder might seem to be emotional disturbance. Unfortunately, the definition of this category in the law (see box "Emotional Disturbance") is vague and lacks a solid grounding in mental health research and practice.

In addition, some parents worry about the potential for bias against students who are labeled as emotionally disturbed. At some schools, teachers may view the label as a synonym for troublemaker. By extension, they may see disruptive behaviors as signs of willful disobedience rather than symptoms of a biologically based disease. At other schools, students labeled as emotionally disturbed may be routed into behavior modification programs that are not necessarily appropriate for teens with a mood disorder. Such programs involve a system of rewards and punishments that are designed to teach appropriate behavior. However, if teens are incapable of responding as intended to the consequences because of unstable moods, this approach may just breed frustration.

For these reasons, some educators advocate that children with mood disorders be placed in a category called "other health impairment" (OHI), which includes attention-deficit hyperactivity disorder as well as other medical illnesses that affect school performance. This classification may reduce the stigma attached to both the students and their family. It may also encourage the school to take biological aspects of depression and bipolar disorder into consideration when making educational or disciplinary decisions. In particular, the OHI label highlights the facts that disruptive behavior related to the mood disorder may not be under a student's control.

The services provided to children under IDEA are based on a written individualized educational plan (IEP), which is described on pp. 140–143. This type of plan allows for needed educational accommodations, ranging from minor modifications in the classroom to placement in a special education class or therapeutic school. The federal government provides extra funding to the schools for students served under IDEA. On the downside, the IEP process can be time-consuming and cumbersome. In addition, some children with mental disorders may not meet the IDEA eligibility criteria.

Section 504 provides another option for such students who attend public schools. It merely requires that students have a

---

### Emotional Disturbance

Below are the IDEA criteria for emotional disturbance:

1. At least one of the following characteristics must be present over a long period of time and to a marked degree that adversely affects a student's educational performance.
   a. An inability to learn that cannot be explained by intellectual, sensory, or health factors
   b. An inability to build or maintain satisfactory interpersonal relationships with peers and teachers
   c. Inappropriate types of behavior or feelings under normal circumstances
   d. A general pervasive mood of unhappiness or depression
   e. A tendency to develop physical symptoms or fears associated with personal or school problems
2. The definition includes schizophrenia.
3. The definition does not include social maladjustment unless it is accompanied by one of the other conditions listed above.

---

### Other Health Impairment

Below are the IDEA criteria for the OHI classification:

1. The student has limited strength or vitality or altered alertness, which results in limited alertness with respect to the educational environment.
2. The cause is a chronic or acute health problem, such as attention-deficit hyperactivity disorder, asthma, diabetes, epilepsy, a heart condition, hemophilia, lead poisoning, leukemia, nephritis, rheumatic fever, or sickle cell anemia.
3. The student's educational performance is adversely affected.

---

physical or mental impairment that substantially limits one or more major life activity—a standard that any student with major depression or bipolar disorder meets. A 504 plan may sometimes provide a more expeditious alternative to an IEP, although it has its own set of requirements. In theory, it can provide for all the same services. However, since schools are not provided additional funding under Section 504 the way they are under IDEA, most prefer not to take the 504 route when extensive accommodations are needed. As a practical matter, some schools may not adhere to a 504 plan as strictly as they do to an IEP, even though there are legal provisions requiring them to do so.

### What Is an IEP, and How Is It Developed?

*a written educational plan for an individual who qualifies for services*

An IEP is a written educational plan for an individual student who qualifies for services under IDEA. The first step in the IEP process is a request for an evaluation, which can be made by school personnel, parents, students, or other interested parties. If you initiate the request, be sure to put it in writing. It's recommended that you either send the letter by certified mail or get a receipt when you hand-deliver it. Once you've made your request, the school must either complete a full evaluation, or give you written notice of its refusal and let you know your rights. Assuming a full evaluation is done, it must be conducted by trained professionals and address all areas related to the suspected disability. The goal is to establish whether the student has a disability that adversely affects his or her ability to perform at school.

You will be notified of the results of the evaluation. If your child is deemed ineligible for services, and you disagree, you can request an independent educational evaluation by an outside party. However, if both you and the school system agree that your child is eligible, the next step is to schedule an IEP team meeting. At this meeting, you, school personnel, and any other team members will develop a plan that is individualized for your child. The team should be willing to consult with your child's doctor or therapist, if appropriate. The plan lists any special services your child needs, goals that your child is expected to achieve in a year, and benchmarks for measuring your child's progress. The IEP team also decides where the services will be provided and what special accommodations may be required. The guiding principle is that a child should be placed in the least restrictive environment possible. This means that your child will not be placed in a self-contained special education class, for example, if his or her needs can be met in a regular classroom.

Assuming you agree with the IEP and proposed placement, you'll sign the IEP, and the plan will be put into effect. You and the rest of the IEP team will then meet at regular intervals to discuss your child's progress, make any needed changes in services, and develop new goals. It's possible that you may not agree with the IEP, however, if you and the other team members are unable to reach a consensus. In that case, don't sign the IEP. To keep the plan from automatically going into effect, you'll need to provide prompt written notice of your disagreement and request another meeting of the IEP team, where you can try to work out a compromise. If that fails, you can then exercise your due process rights as a parent, which include the rights to have input into your child's educational plan and to take action to resolve disputes. You may request an impartial hearing, at which you and the school district are each given a chance to present your case to a hearing officer. Mediation must also be available.

"The goal is never to have to go to due process," says Gilcher. "But from the moment you know your child's diagnosis and seek assistance from the school, you should be preparing your due process complaint, just in case." That means keeping a complete, written record of everything that transpires. Gilcher recommends getting a large, three-ring binder in which to keep copies of:

- Evaluation results
- IEPs
- Medical documents, including ones relating to symptoms of your child's disorder and side effects of your child's medications
- Progress reports or report cards
- Standardized test or proficiency test results
- Written communications, including formal letters and notices, informal notes, and e-mails
- Notes on verbal communications, including phone conversations and face-to-face meetings
- Representative samples of schoolwork

---

### IDEA Reauthorization

At this writing, IDEA is up for reauthorization by Congress. In 2003 and 2004, different versions of a bill reauthorizing the act were passed by the U.S. House and Senate. A joint conference committee will be convened to iron out those differences. Depending on the form of the bill that ultimately is signed into law, certain provisions of IDEA may change. For the latest information, see the websites of the Council for Exceptional Children–IDEA Law and Resources (www.ideapractices.org) and National Dissemination Center for Children with Disabilities (www.nichcy.org).

---

- Financial records, including invoices and receipts, for services you pay for privately to advance your child's education
- Related materials, including information about IDEA and your state's special education policies and procedures

## What Kinds of Accommodations May Be Needed?

Whether your adolescent has an IEP or a 504 plan, certain modifications may be needed to help your teen succeed in the classroom. This is where the individualized part really comes into play, since no two students or classrooms are exactly the same. Following are some examples of modifications that have worked well for other families:

- Self-imposed timeouts—"My daughter has a 'hot pass' that lets her leave the classroom and go to her caseworker whenever she feels like she's about to lose control," says one parent. This gives her daughter an opportunity to prevent blowups before they happen.
- Scheduling adjustments—"I arrange it so my son never has two classes in a row where he has to sit still," says

## Little Changes That Mean a Lot

Gilcher offers these examples of relatively minor modifications that can make a major difference for some students with mood disorders:

*Scheduling*
- Allowing for a later start or a shorter day
- Scheduling the most stimulating classes early in the day to get the student interested
- Scheduling the hardest classes for the time of day when the student is usually most alert

*Instruction*
- Warning students before a change in activities
- Providing movement breaks at regular intervals
- Communicating with parents on a weekly basis about the student's classroom performance
- Allowing a water bottle at the desk
- Permitting frequent bathroom breaks

*Testing*
- Breaking long tests into smaller segments
- Simplifying test instructions
- Allowing extra time for tests
- Providing a test room away from other students and distractions
- Offering other assignments as an alternative to high-stress tests

*Homework*
- Requiring the use of an assignment notebook
- Simplifying homework instructions
- Extending the deadline for big projects

another parent. For instance, her son might follow a math class with PE. Other possible adjustments include starting the school day later or keeping it shorter.

- Alternative assignments—"For my kids, it really helps not to have to give oral presentations in front of the class," says the mother of four students with mood disorders. Instead, students might present material one-on-one to the teacher. Other possible arrangements include simplified instructions for assignments or modified deadlines for homework.

- Outside credit—"My son was in a drug rehab program two hours a day, three days a week. I told the school, 'This is going to help him more in life than any history class or English class.'" The school agreed with this mother and gave her son a high school credit for the program.

It's important for your teen to understand that such modifications aren't a free ride to avoid work or bend rules. "My philosophy is that bipolar disorder isn't an excuse to get out of doing things," says the mother of an eighth grader. "If anything, it means he has to work a little harder." The expectation is that students still need to put forth their personal best effort on any particular day. The school environment is simply adapted to help them make the most of their capabilities.

## Finding Support From Other Parents

Which teachers at your teen's school are most receptive to working with parents? What other easy modifications can help at school or home? And where can you turn when you just need to vent to someone who understands? The best sources of answers for these questions and many more are often other parents of teens with depression and bipolar disorder. Chances are, they've shared many of the same problems as you, and they may have found clever solutions that really work.

*The best sources of answers . . . are often other parents*

When you talk with these parents, you don't have to worry as much about explaining every aspect of your teen's illness or being judged based on misinformation. That isn't always the case with other people. "My son was a wrestler," says one mother. "Before he went into the hospital, I'd go to his practices, and all the parents would talk to me. After he got out of the hospital and went back to wrestling, there was suddenly nobody to talk to. They all went to sit on the other side of the room. I think they just didn't know what to say." Many parents also recount being the targets of mean-spirited gossip or unfair finger-pointing. At times, it can seem tempting just to withdraw into a shell and shut out the rest of the world.

The problem is that this keeps you from utilizing one of the best tools for managing stress: social support. That's why many parents find support and self-help groups so valuable. Such groups offer the benefits of social support in a safe setting, where people understand what you're going through because they're experiencing similar things themselves. In addition, parent groups are often an excellent source of practical advice on handling the day-to-day challenges of raising a teenager with depression or bipolar disorder. And since you can't live in a cocoon all the time, many groups also provide education and advocacy to the public at large. Some lobby the legislators and policymakers who determine what mental health services are available in your community and how students with mental disorders are educated by your schools.

"I started out by joining a support group locally," says one mother-turned-activist. "Since then, I've joined their board of directors, and I'm helping them with programming. I'm also going to run a support group here in my neighborhood. So for me, part of finding support is the creation of support. And it's amazing how many people you meet when you come out of the closet, so to speak, on this issue—how many people will say, my child was just diagnosed, or my nephew or my neighbor. But unless somebody starts the conversation, everyone walks around not talking."

There is no substitute for this kind of face-to-face interaction with other people. However, for parents who are isolated by geography or family demands, online discussion boards, chat rooms, and e-mail lists offer support that can be accessed anywhere, anytime. "When I'm having a bad night, I know I can go to the chat room and talk it out. It's a lifesaver," says one mother. Good starting points for locating both in-person and online support groups include the Depression and Bipolar Support Alliance (DBSA) and the CABF. See the Resources section at the end of this book for complete contact information.

## Chapter Five

# Reducing Risk: Protection and Prevention

Improved diagnosis and treatment may be wonderful, but prevention is much better. Today, some researchers are looking for ways to keep depression and bipolar disorder from starting in the first place. Most scientists now believe that the first episode of a mood disorder may lay down neural pathways within the brain. While these pathways may be modified with medication, psychotherapy, or a combination of both, it's certainly preferable to prevent them from ever forming.

Risk factors are characteristics that increase a person's likelihood of developing an illness. Chapter 2 describes a number of risk factors for depression and bipolar disorder, including a family history of mood disorders, life stress, and family conflict. While these factors may tip the scale toward illness, it's clear that not everyone who has them goes on to develop depression or bipolar disorder. In such cases, protective factors—characteristics that decrease a person's likelihood of developing an illness—may make the critical difference.

Like risk factors, protective factors can potentially be genetic, biological, social, psychological, or behavioral. Some day, we may know more about possible genetic and biological factors that help protect against depression or bipolar disorder. At present, however, most of what we know about the prevention of mood disorders comes from research on social, psychological, and behavioral protective factors. Therefore, this chapter focuses on psychosocial prevention efforts. But it's interesting to speculate about the possibility of biological prevention in the future—

*Some day, we may know more about possible genetic and biological factors that help protect against depression or bipolar disorder.*

for example, a medication that might be taken preventively before the disease has ever developed.

The psychosocial protective factors that researchers are currently studying include individual thinking style and social support. There is still much left to learn. From what we know, however, it's clear that these factors aren't at all like a vaccine that can be applied one time and then counted on to provide nearly total protection for years. Instead, they're more like a diet and exercise plan. For best results, many need to become a regular part of an individual's life. These factors don't confer total immunity against mental illness, either. Nevertheless, the

---

### Prevention 1-2-3

There are three basic types of prevention as it pertains to mental health:

- Primary prevention—Activities that aim to keep the disorder from ever occurring in people who are free of symptoms.
- Secondary prevention—Activities that aim to keep the full-blown disorder from developing in people who have risk factors or early symptoms.
- Tertiary prevention—Activities that aim to reduce the amount of disability associated with an existing disorder or prevent future recurrences.

more protective factors adolescents have going for them, the less likely they may be to ever develop a mood disorder, and the better prepared they may be to cope and recover if they do become ill.

## Developing Optimism and Resilience

Resilience is the ability to adapt well to stressful life events and bounce back from adversity, trauma, or tragedy. Research has shown that optimism is an important element in resilience, and resilience, in turn, tends to bolster hopeful attitudes and positive behavior. As a result, optimism is thought to be an important factor for protecting against the hopelessness of depression. Since depression has multiple causes, optimism alone may not be enough to ward off the illness completely for everyone. However, even in those with a strong biological predisposition to depression, it's possible that optimism might delay the onset or reduce the severity of symptoms.

*Optimism is thought to be an important factor for protecting against the hopelessness of depression*

The Penn Resiliency Program (PRP)—formerly called the Penn Prevention Program—is just one example of a program that strives to build optimism and resiliency in young people. The PRP is a depression prevention curriculum developed especially for middle school students. Based at the University of Pennsylvania, the 14-year-old program targets depression and depressive symptoms, but not bipolar disorder. It is built partly on the work of Martin Seligman, a psychologist who is a pioneer in the study of optimism. The PRP aims to give students the skills they need to combat unrealistically negative thinking, much the way cognitive-behavioral therapy does. But by teaching young people these skills *before* they're seriously depressed, the goal of the program is to stave off depression completely or keep any existing depressive symptoms from getting worse.

As it's currently implemented, the PRP is designed for use by groups of middle school students, with teachers and guidance counselors serving as group leaders. Research on the program has generally been promising. "Across most studies, the program has had a significant effect of either reducing or preventing depressive symptoms in adolescents," says Jane Gillham, the program's codirector. However, because of the methodology used in studies to date, it's still unclear whether that translates into prevention of full-blown major depression.

In one study led by Gillham, the PRP did improve students' explanatory style—the way in which they habitually explain to themselves why events happen. The theory is that people who are pessimistic tend to be more likely to believe that bad events are unchangeable, will undermine everything they do, and are their own fault, rather than the result of chance, circumstance, or the actions of other people. By helping students adopt a less pessimistic explanatory style, Gillham hopes she can increase their resistance to depression. Her research found that students who participated in the PRP did, indeed, have reduced rates of moderate to severe depressive symptoms, compared to a control group of students, for 2 years afterward.

By 3 years, however, this advantage had been lost for reasons that the researchers are still trying to sort out. Also, the researchers measured depressive symptoms, but they didn't evaluate whether individual children met all the diagnostic criteria for major depression. Therefore, it's impossible to say whether the program decreased students' risk of developing the full-fledged disorder.

Recent data indicate the program may have even stronger effects on anxiety than on depression, which perhaps isn't surprising, given the high degree of overlap between the two disorders. Despite the generally good results with both depression and anxiety, however, the PRP is very much a work in progress. For one thing, the program was originally evaluated in schools where the student bodies were mainly White and middle to upper-middle class. Recently, an effort has been made to apply the program to more diverse groups of students. One study that tested the program in two inner-city schools with largely minority student bodies got positive results with Latino students but not with African American students. Another study found positive results with children in Beijing, China. The researchers are currently working to fine-tune the curriculum in order to make it more universally applicable.

---

### When Positive Is Negative

Many adolescents with depression are given to overly pessimistic thinking, in which they're apt to see the dark cloud behind every silver lining. For them, a more accurate explanatory style means learning to identify unrealistically negative thoughts and replace them with more realistically positive ones. However, some teens with bipolar disorder may have the opposite problem during manic episodes. They may have such inflated self-esteem and grandiose ideas about their own abilities that they make wildly inappropriate and often risky choices. In addition, some teens with conduct disorder may be prone to blithely explaining away their behavior, rather than taking responsibility for the hurt or damage they cause. According to Jane Gillham of the Penn Resiliency Program, a reality check for such teens may require looking at the downside, rather than the upside, of their situation. "In the end, what really counts is accuracy," says Gillham. At times, that may mean using the power of negative thinking.

## How Can You Promote Optimism in Your Teen?

One of the latest modifications in the PRP is the addition of parent groups. The students who participate still meet in their own group after school, but a separate group for parents also is held in the evening. This phase of the program is still in its infancy, so no results are available yet to show whether the parent group really makes a difference over and above the benefits provided by the student program. However, Gillham expects that the parent group may help in at least two ways. For one thing, "it may undercut depression in parents, which is itself a risk factor for depression in kids," she says. "Plus, if we can teach parents to think more accurately and less pessimistically, then they can provide good role models for their students at home."

With or without this kind of formal instruction, Gillham believes that parents can have a positive influence on their teens by becoming aware of their own explanatory style and making an effort to vocalize more realistic thinking. "When you catch yourself jumping to a conclusion, point it out," she suggests. Then talk yourself through the process of evaluating not only the worst case scenario but also the best case and most likely case. Children often learn by imitating those they admire. By modeling the process of evaluating your own thinking, weighing the evidence, and correcting the inaccuracies, you can help them learn these essential skills.

*"When you catch yourself jumping to a conclusion, point it out"*

Later, if your teen shares a thought that seems skewed by overly pessimistic thinking, you can gently guide him or her through the evaluation process. Let's say your teen is talking about a temporary problem as if it will never end. "You might say, 'I know this is really hard right now, but let's think about

# More Prevention Programs

Following is a sampling of other prevention programs from around the world that have targeted depression or depressive symptoms in adolescents.

- Problem Solving for Life, Australia—This 8-week program taught students cognitive techniques for identifying and challenging irrationally negative thoughts as well as skills for solving everyday problems. In a study of 1,500 eighth-graders, the program decreased depressive symptoms between the beginning of the program and the end, but only for students who started out with "high risk" scores on a depression test. Unfortunately, a year later, there was no difference in the rate of diagnosed depression between high-risk students who had taken part in the program and those who hadn't.

- Thoughts and Health, Iceland—This was a cognitive and behavioral program designed to prevent depression. In a study of 72 students at risk for major depression, about half were randomly assigned to take part in the program, while the other were assigned to a control group that did not participate in the program. At the end of the program, there were no differences between the two groups in depressive symptoms or cognitive style. However, 6 months later, 18% of those in the control group had developed major depression or dysthymia, compared to only 3% of the program participants.

- Preventive Intervention Project, Boston—This research targeted children, ages 8 to 15, who had a parent with a mood disorder. Children of such parents have an increased risk of developing depression and other emotional problems themselves. In a study of 93 families, participants were randomly assigned to either attend two parents-only lectures or take part in a 6- to 11-session program that included separate meetings for parents and children. In both the lectures and the meetings, information was shared about the nature of mood disorders and ways of building resilience in children. Two and a half years later, children in both groups still reported having a better understanding of their parent's illness due to the program. The researchers hypothesize that enhanced understanding of the parent's mood disorder may lead to greater self-understanding, which, in turn, may promote increased resilience in the children.

how you've gotten through similar situations before,'" says Gillham. Or if your teen is unrealistically expecting the worst, "you might say, 'Let's think about what evidence there is that this horrible thing you're imagining is actually going to happen.'"

## How Else Can You Encourage Resilience?

Instilling an optimistic attitude is just one part of building resilience. There are a number of other things you can do to help your adolescent develop skills for coping more effectively with the hardships and letdowns that are an inevitable part of growing up:

- Spend time together as a family. One recent survey of over 4,700 adolescents found that something as simple as sharing family meals can reduce the risk of depressive symptoms and suicidal thoughts or behaviors. In today's time-stressed families, however, such everyday rituals can easily fall by the wayside. The same survey found that only about one-quarter of adolescents said they had shared at least seven meals with all or most of their family over the past week. Make a conscious effort to set aside time to spend with your teen every day.

  *Spend time together as a family.*

- Help your teen connect with others. A strong network of extended family and friends can bolster your teen's social skills and provide additional sources of emotional support through good times and bad. "We redid the basement so the kids could come to my house and hang out," says one mother. "I always have a gang of boys in my basement! And I'm always feeding them and buying cases of soda. But I wanted my son and his friends to feel comfortable here."

- Nurture your teen's self-esteem. Considering all the changes and challenges facing teenagers, it's not surprising that the teen years are often fraught with self-doubt. Remind your adolescent of times when he or she has dealt with a challenge successfully. Then help your teen see that even past setbacks are part of a growth process that builds strength and teaches skills, making it easier to handle the next challenge that comes along.
- Encourage hobbies and interests. Positive activities give adolescents a chance to develop their talents and abilities, stimulate their minds, and engage their enthusiasm. Many activities provide other benefits as well. For example, participation in a sport may enhance physical health and teach teamwork, while volunteering for a cause may instill altruism and social awareness. Allow plenty of time for less structured activities, too. Promote active self-discovery by encouraging your adolescent to spend some quiet time writing in a journal, playing music, drawing and painting, building models, caring for a pet—whatever your teen enjoys.
- Teach stress management skills. Stress is an unavoidable part of life. You can't shelter your teen from all stress, but you can help him or her learn to keep it from spiraling out of control. Make sure that your teen's life isn't overscheduled; downtime is just as important as soccer practice and piano lessons. Encourage the use of simple stress reduction techniques, such as deep breathing, exercise, and short self-imposed timeouts. Then be a good role model by making relaxation a regular part of your day as well.
- Provide a stress-free zone. Ideally, home should be a haven from the pressures of the outside world. Try to create

## "I Can Do It!"

Self-efficacy is the formal term for people's beliefs about their own ability to perform effectively in a particular situation. People with high self-efficacy believe in their capability to achieve the results they want through their own efforts. The concept is closely linked to hope and optimism. Not surprisingly, a high sense of self-efficacy has been associated with a decreased risk of depression in young people. Parents may not toss around words like "self-efficacy" in casual conversation, but many seem to know on an instinctual level how to build it.

- Help your teen develop valued skills, step by step. "When he started to a new high school, he wanted to begin driving himself," says one mother. "I drove him every day at first until he was comfortable with the route. Then he drove himself, and I followed in my car until he got comfortable with that. And then finally, he was ready to go on his own."

- Set your teen up for success. "Jason went to camp for the first time this summer," says the mother of a 14-year-old. "Our social worker's daughters go to the same camp, so she called the director up, and the director met with us in the social worker's office to go over expectations." While Jason was at camp, the staff administered his medication, and they lent a hand when he had trouble getting along with another camper. "Jason couldn't call home for the whole month, but he had the option to call the social worker if he needed to. He never called. And he loved it so much he was sad to come home."

a home environment that feels safe, secure, and structured for predictability and consistency. Realistically, though, most families go through periods when the stability of the home routine temporarily breaks down. At such times, it's more important than ever that your child still has a place to unwind and decompress.

Sharlene, the mother of three, is a firm believer in this last point. Her teenage daughter and son have bipolar disorder, while her 10-year-old son has not shown any symptoms. She thinks that her younger son has especially benefited from having a getaway spot to temporarily escape when family tensions come to a boil. "Fortunately, he's able to have his own bedroom," says Sharlene. "He needs his own space when there's turmoil with the other ones. You have to make sure the one who doesn't have issues gets his needs met, too. You have to make sure he's got his own space." Just be careful that your child doesn't start shutting everyone out completely. The idea is to offer a temporary refuge from stress and strife, not promote withdrawal.

## Reducing Family Risk Factors

Along with promoting the positives in your adolescent's life, you can work to remove as many negatives as possible. Some risk factors, such as a genetic predisposition to mood disorders or a traumatic event that occurred in the past, can't be changed. However, others can be eliminated or controlled, and it makes sense to address these factors proactively. If your teen has already developed a mood disorder, you may be able to decrease symptoms or head off a recurrence in the future.

Researchers are just starting to pinpoint the many risk factors for adolescent mood disorders. Some of these have to do with family interactions and the home environment. This doesn't mean that parents directly cause mood disorders in their teens. But it does mean that parents may be able to take steps to reduce some risk factors and possibly minimize problems. Based on the research to date, these are some known risk factors for depression that can be eliminated or changed:

- Lack of emotional closeness and support within the family
- A family life characterized by constant fighting and conflict

- Domestic violence or child abuse
- Untreated depression in the parents
- Parental alcohol or drug abuse

Remember that there are numerous other influences acting on your adolescent, including genetic and biological factors that aren't under either your or your teen's control. Changing family risk factors won't necessarily prevent your teen from developing a mood disorder. However, a calmer, more stable home life will certainly give your teen a stronger base from which to meet life's challenges. And if your adolescent does develop depression or bipolar disorder, a supportive family can make a big difference in how well your teen responds to treatment. At the same time, warm family relationships may help protect your teen from developing other problems that sometimes go along with depression or bipolar disorder, such as substance abuse.

If you recognize any of the risk factors listed above in your own family, now is the time to seek help. Individual or family counseling may help you better manage your own feelings and make positive changes in your life. For one father, the crucial lesson he learned was how to better control his temper:

"One of the things I've learned—and this is probably a good parenting rule in any circumstance—is to try not to react viscerally when something happens with the kids. I need to just stop and think for a minute, and try to sort out what's going on before reacting. There were many, many occasions with my children when they did something that I thought was out of line, and I reacted with anger and some sort of extreme discipline.

I look back now, and I don't understand why I had such a strong reaction at the time. I'm still learning, but I'm making a real effort to look at things and provide a more appropriate

*"I need to just stop and think for a minute, and try to sort out what's going on before reacting."*

response. Rather than too firm a hand, on one hand, or too much sympathy and acceptance of unacceptable behavior, on the other, I'm trying to find the middle ground."

## Dos and Don'ts of Resolving Conflicts

*Do . . .*

- pick your battles. Avoid getting into arguments over issues that aren't worth the emotional wear and tear.
- take some deep breaths, count to 10, or excuse yourself for a couple of minutes to calm down if you're angry.
- use humor to defuse a tense situation. Just make sure it isn't an angry or sarcastic remark disguised as a "joke."
- realize that the hurtful things your teen says during an argument aren't really about you. They're about your teen's need to learn to handle strong emotions.
- talk about the situation once you've both cooled off. State the problem and explain your perspective calmly.
- ask your teen to share his or her thoughts on the matter. Give your teen's viewpoint careful consideration.
- look for a compromise solution, if possible. When you need to assert your authority, be calm but firm.

*Don't . . .*

- expect a teen in the grips of a depressive or manic episode to be very receptive to reasoning until his or her mood is better stabilized.
- let anger become a habit in your family. If conflict gets to be a frequent or severe problem, seek help from a mental health professional.

## Preventing Suicide

For adolescents who have already developed depression or bipolar disorder, one important goal of prevention efforts is to prevent suicide. Many depression-related suicides occur during the first few episodes of illness, before a person has learned that the hopeless feelings and suicidal thoughts will eventually pass. This is one reason why adolescents, who don't yet have much life experience dealing with their symptoms, may be at risk for acting on their suicidal impulses.

Just as for depression and bipolar disorder, there are protective factors and risk factors for suicide. Research has shown that one of the strongest protective factors for young people is having a family that is emotionally supportive and involved. A feeling of connectedness to school also seems to be protective. In addition, it has been suggested that good problem-solving skills may reduce the risk of suicidal behavior. Although the latter link hasn't been definitely proven, it stands to reason that teens who are able to think through difficult problems and come up with workable solutions might be less likely to see suicide as their only option.

> Good problem-solving skills may reduce the risk of suicidal behavior.

To help your adolescent become an effective problem solver, first help him or her define the problem at hand. Then brainstorm together about possible solutions. Next, consider the pros and cons of each solution in turn, until your teen can choose the best solution for the situation. Finally, develop a plan for putting that solution into action. By walking your adolescent through this process, you're teaching an essential life skill that may help your teen make more positive choices.

## How Can You Reduce the Risk of Suicide?

As far as risk factors for suicide go, a large majority of adolescents who die by suicide have serious mental health conditions, such as depression, bipolar disorder, substance abuse, conduct disorder, or oppositional defiant disorder. A personal history of past suicidal behavior is also a strong predictor of both subsequent suicide attempts and death by suicide. This relationship is especially evident among young people with depression and bipolar disorder. Therefore, one of the most effective ways of reducing the risk of suicide is by getting your adolescent prompt, professional treatment for depression, mania, substance abuse, or other mental health problems as they arise.

Another factor influencing the likelihood of death by suicide is easy access to highly lethal methods, particularly firearms. Recent studies have found that the odds of a young person dying by suicide are many times higher in homes where guns are present than in homes without guns. It's noteworthy that young people who use firearms for suicide tend to have fewer warning signs leading up to their deaths—such as mental illness, substance abuse, or suicidal talk—than those who use other methods. Thus, it seems that suicide by gunshot may often be an impulsive act dependent on ready access to a gun. The most cautious approach is not to keep firearms in your home, especially if there is an adolescent with a mental health issue in the household. But if you choose to have firearms, any gun should always be kept locked up and unloaded.

Young people also seem to be particularly vulnerable to "suicide contagion"—in other words, an increase in suicidal thoughts and behavior upon learning about the suicide of a friend or family member, a celebrity, or even a total stranger whose death is reported by the media. The fictional portrayal of suicide in a movie or on television may also increase the risk in susceptible teens. When suicide comes up in any context, discuss it honestly with your adolescent. For example, if you've just watched a movie together in which a character died by suicide, strike up a conversation

*When suicide comes up in any context, discuss it honestly with your adolescent.*

afterward about other steps the character could have taken in response to his or her problem. In addition to starting a dialogue about the movie, use this opportunity to let your teen know that suicide is a topic the two of you can discuss.

Stressful life events may also be associated with suicide in young people who are already at risk because of mental illness or substance abuse. Among the more common triggers for youth suicide are an argument with a parent, a romantic breakup, bullying, school problems, or trouble with the law. In times of stress, be especially alert for warning signs of possible suicidal thoughts. As always, get help immediately if you suspect that your teen may be thinking about suicide.

One last factor that may be associated with youth suicide is homosexuality. Several studies have found an increased rate of attempted suicide among adolescents with this sexual orientation, whether or not they have actually had sexual contact yet. A number of possible reasons for the link have been proposed, including stigma, bullying and teasing, social isolation, and parental rejection. For adolescents who are struggling to come to terms with their sexuality at the same time that they're dealing with a mood disorder, the pressure can be especially intense.

"My son came out his sophomore year of high school," says the mother of Tom, who has bipolar disorder. "He was teased horribly. They yelled names at him as he walked down the hall. One social worker actually said to me, 'Well, if he's going to flame, he deserves it.' Can you believe it?" The pressure at school became so unbearable that Tom was ready to drop out. Not surprisingly, this was also a period when Tom had considerable difficulty keeping his symptoms in check.

Ultimately, Tom was placed in a special school that was intended primarily for youngsters with conduct problems. "And there he was, this sweet kid who just wasn't going to school anymore because he couldn't stand the teasing," his mother says. "Nothing special was done for him. The bipolar meant nothing. There was no recognition that maybe he would have more difficulty than the next kid."

Despite the challenges, Tom made it through high school—if not exactly unscathed, then at least stronger for having survived the experience. Part of the credit undoubtedly goes to his mother, who was unwavering in her emotional support.

*You can offer the unconditional love and acceptance that help your teen develop resilience and a sense of self-worth.*

The moral: You may not be able to shield your adolescent from every cruel barb, but you can offer the unconditional love and acceptance that help your teen develop resilience and a sense of self-worth. If your teen has depression or bipolar disorder, you can also provide appropriate treatment. These two factors combined may often make the critical difference for adolescents who might otherwise be vulnerable to suicide.

## Looking at the Big Picture: Prevention at the Societal Level

In addition to all the positive things you can do on an individual level as a parent, researchers are trying to find ways to combat depression, bipolar disorder, and suicide at the societal level. The PRP is an example of this kind of prevention program. It's designed to be a universal intervention, which is a program intended to benefit an entire group of people, not just those identified as being at risk. The main goal of this kind of program is a reduction in the occurrence of new cases of a disorder.

Some other programs are selective interventions, which target a particular subgroup of individuals who have a higher-than-average risk of developing the disorder. Biological, psychological, or social risk factors may be used to identify those who qualify for this type of program. Still other programs are indicated interventions, which target individuals who have some symptoms of the disorder but don't yet meet all the diagnostic criteria for the full-fledged illness.

Whatever the target audience, most programs aimed at preventing depression take an approach similar to that of the PRP. They use cognitive-behavioral techniques and family education to reduce risk factors and enhance protective factors and resilience. The results so far have been encouraging. However, considerably more research is still needed. Several key questions remain to be answered, such as the most effective components to include in these programs and the best age to present them. We also need to learn more about how to make the programs more relevant to young people from diverse racial, ethnic, and socioeconomic backgrounds.

Nevertheless, the potential to help program participants seems clear. In Oregon, for example, Gregory Clarke and his colleagues developed a program they called the Adolescent Coping With Stress course. The course consisted of 15 after-school group meetings held over a 5-week period. It emphasized teaching cognitive-behavioral coping skills. In one study of 150 ninth- and tenth-graders, students who took part in the program were less likely than a control group to be diagnosed with major depression or dysthymia during the following year. Since about one-third of the program participants had already suffered from depression in the past, the program may have helped prevent not only first episodes of depression but also relapses or recurrences.

The payoffs of such programs for society could be substantial. For one thing, they might reduce the cost of treating not only mood disorders but also associated conditions such as substance abuse. They might also decrease the need for special education as well as other support services for adolescents with mood disorders and their families. In addition, they might relieve the burden on juvenile justice and child welfare agencies, which are often inappropriately tapped to deal with mentally ill adolescents.

Given the many potential benefits for both individual adolescents and society, it's unfortunate that prevention programs aren't more widely available. To a large extent, this is due to lack of research, and that, in turn, is due to inadequate funding. As a parent, you can become an advocate on behalf of greater funding in this area. Write your government representatives, and let them know that research on adolescent mental health is a priority for you. It's one more way in which you can make a difference in the lives of your adolescent and all the young people in your community and society at large.

*As a parent, you can become an advocate on behalf of greater funding in this area.*

## Chapter Six

# Conclusion: Take Action, Take Heart

No one has a bigger stake in ongoing research on the diagnosis, treatment, management, and prevention of mood disorders than you. As the parent of an adolescent with depression or bipolar disorder, you are directly affected by any new advances that such research might bring. There is an urgency and immediacy to your concern, since the drive to protect and nurture your child is a powerful, primal force. You can draw on that energy to become an agent for change, both in the private life of your adolescent and in the public realm of American society.

> The drive to protect and nurture your child is a powerful, primal force . . . draw on that energy to become an agent for change.

Several of the parents quoted in the earlier pages of this book have become outspoken advocates for young people with depression and bipolar disorder. Each has found his or her individual way to make a mark. Some have worked as volunteers or paid staff for support and advocacy organizations. Others have written letters to politicians and policymakers. Still others have frequently made themselves available to the media for interviews. And all, of course, were willing to share their stories in this book.

Some parents found creative ways to use their unique skills to educate others. For example, a few wrote about their experiences for publication. And one mother, a social worker at a state mental health facility, teamed up with her teenage daughter to give a talk about bipolar disorder to the social work department there. "She talked about her experiences, and I had handouts about it," says Lynn. "I gave a little presentation, and then they asked her questions." Lynn notes that she only took this route once it became clear that her daughter was eager to participate. "I decided to do this with her, not to exploit her, but so she would learn to speak out and not feel stigmatized." In the process, the social workers at this particular facility gained a richer understanding of bipolar disorder that will doubtless carry over into their work with other teens.

If your adolescent, like Lynn's daughter, wants to reach out to others about mental health issues, help your teen find meaningful ways of doing this. Of course, you shouldn't pressure your teen to do anything that doesn't feel comfortable. Many teens, however, welcome the chance to advocate on their own behalf. After all, it's their future at stake.

Taken together, all these small steps can add up to substantial progress. To get the forward momentum started in your community, share information and resources with those who have an impact on young people, such as teachers, primary care physicians, sports coaches, youth group leaders, and directors of local social service organizations. Get involved in support and advocacy groups, and volunteer your time and energy in whatever way seems most appropriate for you.

## Things *Will* Get Better

Of all the suggestions and insights these parents wanted to share, the one they emphasized most was a simple but powerful message: *Don't give up!* Parenting a teen with depression or bipolar disorder can be a long and arduous task. With time and appropriate treatment, however, there's an excellent chance your adolescent's mood will stabilize, and his or her symptoms will improve. As your teen's prospects brighten, your own life will get easier. There is an end in sight.

> "We've been through the turmoil, and I think we've finally seen the light," says Sharlene. "But there were 6 or 7 years there where I didn't know if we were ever going to get out of it. I think the most important thing is not to give up on them. When things were at their worst, I told myself, 'If they have to go through these things in their life, at least they're at home where I can help them with it.' And I looked at it as a challenge and a blessing that I could help them get through the bad times."

# Glossary

**acute treatment**   Any treatment that is aimed at achieving remission of symptoms.

**adrenal glands**   Glands located just above the kidneys. Their hormones help regulate many physiological functions, including the body's stress response.

**adrenocorticotropic hormone (ACTH)**   A hormone released by the pituitary gland.

**anticipation**   A genetic pattern in which there is a tendency for individuals in successive generations to develop hereditary disorders at earlier ages and with more severe symptoms.

**anticonvulsant**   A medication that helps prevent seizures. Many anticonvulsants have mood-stabilizing effects as well.

**antidepressant**   A medication used to prevent or relieve depression.

**antipsychotic**   A medication used to prevent or relieve psychotic symptoms. Some newer antipsychotics have mood-stabilizing effects as well.

**anxiety disorder**   Any of several mental disorders that are characterized by extreme or maladaptive feelings of tension, fear, or worry.

**attention-deficit hyperactivity disorder (ADHD)**   A disorder characterized by a short attention span, excessive activity, or impulsive behavior. The symptoms of the disorder begin early in life.

**atypical antipsychotic**   One of the newer antipsychotic medications. Some atypical antipsychotics are also used as mood stabilizers.

**atypical depression**   A form of major depression or dysthymia in which the person is able to cheer up when something good happens, but then sinks back into depression once the positive event has passed.

**axon**    The sending branch on a nerve cell.

**bipolar disorder not otherwise specified (BP-NOS)**    A term used for any form of bipolar disorder that doesn't meet the diagnostic criteria for bipolar I, bipolar II, or cyclothymia.

**bipolar disorder**    A mood disorder characterized by an overly high mood, called mania, which alternates with depression.

**bipolar I disorder**    A form of bipolar disorder characterized by the occurrence of at least one manic or mixed episode, often preceded by an episode of major depression.

**bipolar II disorder**    A form of bipolar disorder characterized by an alternating pattern of hypomania and major depression.

**catatonia**    A state of severely disordered activity characterized by physical immobility, purposeless overactivity, extreme negativism, refusal to speak, parrot-like echoing of someone else's words, or mimicking of another's movements.

**chronic depression**    A form of major depression in which symptoms are present continuously for at least 2 years.

**clinical psychologist**    A mental health professional who provides assessment and therapy for mental and emotional disorders.

**cognitive-behavioral therapy (CBT)**    A form of psychotherapy that aims to correct ingrained patterns of thinking and behavior that may be contributing to a person's mental, emotional, or behavioral symptoms.

**comorbidity**    The simultaneous presence of two or more disorders.

**conduct disorder**    A disorder characterized by a repetitive or persistent pattern of having extreme difficulty following rules or conforming to social norms.

**continuation therapy**    Any treatment that is aimed at preventing a relapse.

**corticotropin-releasing factor (CRF)**    A substance released by the hypothalamus.

**cortisol**    A hormone released by the adrenal glands that is responsible for many of the physiological effects of stress.

**crisis residential treatment services**    Temporary, 24-hour care in a nonhospital setting during a crisis.

**cyclothymia**    A mood disorder characterized by cycling between hypomania and relatively mild depressive symptoms. This pattern lasts for at least a year, and any intermittent periods of normal mood last no longer than 2 months at a time.

**day treatment**    See partial hospitalization.

**delusion**    A bizarre belief that is seriously out of touch with reality.

**depression**   A feeling of being sad, hopeless, or apathetic that lasts for at least a couple of weeks. See major depression.

***Diagnostic and Statistical Manual of Mental Disorders,* Fourth Edition, Text Revision (*DSM-IV-TR*)**   A manual that mental health professionals use for diagnosing all kinds of mental illnesses.

**dopamine**   A neurotransmitter that is essential for movement and also influences motivation and perception of reality.

**dysthymia**   A mood disorder that involves being either mildly depressed or irritable most of the day. These feelings occur more days than not for 12 months or longer and are associated with other symptoms.

**eating disorder**   A disorder characterized by serious disturbances in eating behavior. People may severely restrict what they eat, or they may go on eating binges, then attempt to compensate by such means as self-induced vomiting or misuse of laxatives.

**electroconvulsive therapy (ECT)**   A treatment that involves delivering a carefully controlled electrical current to the brain, which produces a brief seizure. This is thought to alter some of the electrochemical processes involved in brain functioning.

**endorphins**   Protein-like compounds in the brain that have natural pain-relieving and mood-elevating effects.

**explanatory style**   The way in which people habitually explain to themselves why events happen.

**family therapy**   Psychotherapy that brings together several members of a family for therapy sessions.

**frontal lobes**   Part of the brain involved in planning, reasoning, controlling voluntary movement, and turning thoughts into words.

**gamma-amino-butyric acid (GABA)**   A neurotransmitter that inhibits the flow of nerve signals in neurons by blocking the release of other neurotransmitters.

**group therapy**   Psychotherapy that brings together several patients with similar diagnoses or issues for therapy sessions.

**hallucination**   The sensory perception of something that isn't really there.

**health maintenance organization (HMO)**   A type of managed care plan in which members must use health care providers who work for the HMO.

**hippocampus**   Part of the brain that plays a role in learning, memory, and emotion.

**home-based services**   Assistance provided in a patient's home to improve family coping skills and avert the need for more intensive services.

**hospitalization**    Inpatient treatment in a facility that provides intensive, specialized care and close, round-the-clock monitoring.

**hypomania**    A somewhat high, expansive, or irritable mood that lasts for at least 4 days. The mood is more moderate than with mania, but also clearly different from a person's usual mood when not depressed.

**hypothalamic-pituitary-adrenal (HPA) axis**    A body system comprised of the hypothalamus, pituitary gland, and adrenal glands along with the substances these structures secrete.

**hypothalamus**    Part of the brain that serves as the command center for the nervous and hormonal systems.

**indicated prevention program**    A program that targets individuals who have some symptoms of a disorder but don't yet meet all the diagnostic criteria for the full-fledged illness.

**individual therapy**    Psychotherapy in which a patient meets one-on-one with a therapist.

**individualized educational plan (IEP)**    A written educational plan for an individual student who qualifies for services under IDEA.

**Individuals with Disabilities Education Act (IDEA)**    A federal law that applies to students who have a disability that impacts their ability to benefit from general educational services.

**interpersonal therapy (IPT)**    A form of psychotherapy that aims to address the interpersonal triggers for mental, emotional, or behavioral symptoms.

**Katie Beckett option**    See TEFRA option.

**kindling hypothesis**    A theory stating that repeated episodes of mania or depression may spark long-lasting changes in the brain, making it more sensitive to future stress.

**learning disorder**    A disorder that adversely affects a person's performance in school or ability to function in everyday situations that require reading, writing, or math skills.

**light therapy**    A therapeutic regimen of daily exposure to very bright light from an artificial source.

**lithium**    A mood-stabilizing medication.

**maintenance therapy**    Any treatment that is aimed at preventing a recurrence of symptoms.

**major depression**    A mood disorder that involves either being depressed or irritable nearly all time, or losing interest or enjoyment in almost everything. These feelings last for at least 2 weeks, are associated with several other symptoms, and cause significant distress or impaired functioning.

**managed care**    A system for controlling health care costs.

**mania**    An overly high or irritable mood that lasts for at least a week or leads to dangerous behavior. Symptoms include grandiose ideas, decreased need for sleep, racing thoughts, risk taking, and increased talking or activity. These symptoms cause marked impairment in functioning or relationships.

**manic depression**    See bipolar disorder.

**Medicaid**    A government program, paid for by a combination of federal and state funds, that provides health and mental health care to low-income individuals who meet eligibility criteria.

**medical necessity**    A standard used by managed care plans in determining whether or not to pay for a health care service. To satisfy this standard, the service must be deemed medically appropriate and necessary to meet a patient's health care needs.

**melancholia**    A severe form of major depression in which there is a near-complete absence of interest or pleasure in anything.

**melatonin**    A hormone that regulates the body's internal clock, which controls daily rhythms of sleep, body temperature, and hormone secretion.

**mental health parity**    A policy that attempts to equalize the way that mental and physical illnesses are covered by health plans.

**mental illness**    A mental disorder that is characterized by abnormalities in mood, emotion, thought, or higher-order behaviors, such as social interaction or the planning of future activities.

**minor depression**    A term sometimes used to describe a depressive episode that is similar to major depression but involves fewer symptoms and less impairment in everyday functioning.

**mixed episode**    A bipolar episode that is characterized by a mixture of mania and depression occurring at the same time.

**monoamine oxidase inhibitor (MAOI)**    An older class of antidepressant.

**mood disorder**    A mental disorder in which a disturbance in mood is the chief feature.

**mood stabilizer**    A medication for bipolar disorder that reduces manic and/or depressive symptoms and helps even out mood swings.

**mood**    A pervasive emotion that colors a person's whole view of the world.

**neuron**    A cell in the brain or another part of the nervous system that is specialized to send, receive, and process information.

**neurotransmitter**    A chemical that acts as a messenger within the brain.

**norepinephrine**    A neurotransmitter that plays a role in the body's response to stress and helps regulate arousal, sleep, and blood pressure.

**oppositional defiant disorder**   A disorder characterized by a persistent pattern of unusually frequent defiance, hostility, or lack of cooperation.

**partial hospitalization**   Services such as individual and group therapy, special education, vocational training, parent counseling, and therapeutic recreational activities that are provided for at least 4 hours per day.

**phototherapy**   See light therapy.

**pituitary gland**   A small gland located at the base of the brain. Its hormones control other glands and help regulate growth, metabolism, and reproduction.

**placebo**   A sugar pill that looks like a real medication, but does not contain an active ingredient.

**point of service (POS) plan**   A type of managed care plan that is similar to a traditional HMO or PPO, except that members can also use providers outside the HMO organization or PPO network in exchange for a higher copayment or deductible.

**postpartum depression**   A form of major depression in which the symptoms begin within 4 weeks of giving birth.

**preferred provider organization (PPO)**   A type of managed care plan in which members may choose from a network of providers who have contracts with the PPO.

**prefrontal cortex**   Part of the brain involved in complex thought, problem solving, and emotion.

**primary prevention**   Activities that aim to keep a disorder from ever occurring in people who are free of symptoms.

**protective factor**   A characteristic that decreases a person's likelihood of developing an illness.

**psychiatrist**   A medical doctor who specializes in the diagnosis and treatment of mental illnesses and emotional problems.

**psychosis**   A state of severely disordered thinking characterized by delusions or hallucinations.

**psychotherapy**   The treatment of a mental, emotional, or behavioral disorder through "talk therapy" and other psychological techniques.

**randomized controlled trial**   A study in which participants are randomly assigned to a treatment group or a control group. The control group receives either a placebo or standard care. This study design allows researchers to determine which changes in the treatment group over time are due to the treatment itself.

**rapid cycling bipolar disorder**   A form of bipolar disorder in which four or more mood episodes occur within a single year.

**receptor**   A molecule that recognizes a specific chemical, such as a neurotransmitter. For a chemical message to be sent from one nerve cell to another, the message must be delivered to a matching receptor on the surface of the receiving nerve cell.

**recurrence**   A repeat episode of an illness.

**relapse**   The re-emergence of symptoms after a period of remission.

**remission**   A return to the level of functioning that existed before an illness.

**residential treatment center**   A facility that provides round-the-clock supervision and care in a dorm-like group setting. The treatment is less specialized and intensive than in a hospital, but the length of stay is often considerably longer.

**resilience**   The ability to adapt well to stressful life events and bounce back from adversity, trauma, or tragedy.

**respite care**   Child care provided by trained parents or mental health aides to give the usual caregivers a short break.

**reuptake**   The process by which a neurotransmitter is absorbed back into the sending branch of the nerve cell that originally released it.

**risk factor**   A characteristic that increases a person's likelihood of developing an illness.

**S-adenosyl-L-methionine (SAM-e)**   A natural compound that is sold as a dietary supplement.

**schizoaffective disorder**   A severe form of mental illness in which an episode of either depression or mania occurs at the same time as symptoms of schizophrenia.

**schizophrenia**   A severe form of mental illness characterized by delusions, hallucinations, or serious disturbances in speech, behavior, or emotion.

**seasonal affective disorder (SAD)**   A form of major depression in which the symptoms start and stop around the same time each year. Typically, they begin in the fall or winter and subside in the spring. Also called seasonal depression.

**second messenger**   A molecule inside a nerve cell that lets certain parts of the cell know when a specific receptor has been activated by a neurotransmitter.

**secondary prevention**   Activities that aim to keep the full-blown disorder from developing in people who have risk factors or early symptoms.

**Section 504**   students who have a physical and mental impairment that substantially limits one or more major life activities.

**selective prevention program**   A program that targets a particular subgroup of individuals who have a higher-than-average risk of developing a disorder.

**selective serotonin reuptake inhibitor (SSRI)**   A widely prescribed class of antidepressant.

**self-efficacy**   The belief in one's own ability to perform effectively in a particular situation.

**serotonin**   A neurotransmitter that plays a role in mood and helps regulate sleep, appetite, and sexual drive.

**side effect**   An unintended effect of a drug.

**social rhythm therapy**   A therapeutic technique that focuses on helping people regularize their daily routines.

**St. John's wort** (*Hypericum perforatum*)   An herb that is sold as a dietary supplement.

**State Child Health Insurance Program (SCHIP)**   A government program that provides insurance coverage for children whose families have an income level that is slightly above the cutoff for Medicaid eligibility.

**stress response**   The physiological response to any perceived threat—real or imagined, physical or psychological.

**substance abuse**   The continued use of alcohol or other drugs despite negative consequences, such as dangerous behavior while under the influence or substance-related personal, social, or legal problems.

**suicidality**   Suicidal thinking or behavior.

**switching**   The rapid transition from depression to hypomania or mania.

**synapse**   The gap that separates nerve cells.

**system of care**   A network of mental health and social services that are organized to work together to provide care for a particular patient and his or her family.

**TEFRA option**   A funding option, authorized by the Tax Equity and Financial Responsibility Act of 1982, that allows states to provide community- and home-based services for children with disabilities who are living at home and need extensive care.

**temperament**   A person's inborn tendency to react to events in a particular way.

**tertiary prevention**   Activities that aim to reduce the amount of disability associated with an existing disorder or prevent future recurrences.

**transcranial magnetic stimulation (TMS)**   An experimental treatment in which a special electromagnet is placed near the scalp, where it can be used to deliver short bursts of energy to stimulate the nerve cells in a specific part of the brain.

**transporter**   A molecule that carries a chemical messenger, called a neurotransmitter, back to the nerve cell that originally sent the message.

**tricyclic antidepressant (TCA)**   An older class of antidepressant.

**universal prevention program**   A program intended to benefit an entire group of people, not just those identified as being at risk for developing a disorder.

**utilization review**   A formal review of health care services by a managed care plan to determine whether payment for them should be authorized or denied.

**vagus nerve stimulation (VNS)**   An epilepsy treatment that is currently being tested for severe, hard-to-treat depression. It uses a small implanted device to deliver mild electrical pulses to the vagus nerve, which connects to key parts of the brain.

# Resources

## Organizations

American Academy of Child and Adolescent Psychiatry
3615 Wisconsin Avenue NW
Washington, DC 20016-3007
(202) 966-7300
www.aacap.org

American Association of Suicidology
4201 Connecticut Avenue N.W., Suite 408
Washington, DC 20008
(202) 237-2280
www.suicidology.org

American Foundation for Suicide Prevention
120 Wall Street, 22nd Floor
New York, NY 10005
(888) 333-2377
www.afsp.org

American Psychiatric Association
1000 Wilson Boulevard, Suite 1825
Arlington, VA 22209-3901
(703) 907-7300
www.psych.org

American Psychological Association
750 First Street NE
Washington, DC 20002-4242
(800) 374-2721
www.apa.org

Bazelon Center for Mental Health Law
1101 15th Street NW, Suite 1212
Washington, DC 20005
(202) 467-5730
www.bazelon.org

Child and Adolescent Bipolar Foundation
1187 Wilmette Avenue, PMB 331
Wilmette, IL 60091
(847) 256-8525
www.cabf.org

Council for Exceptional Children
1110 N. Glebe Road, Suite 300
Arlington, VA 22201
(703) 620-3660
www.cec.sped.org

Depression and Bipolar Support Alliance
730 N. Franklin Street, Suite 501
Chicago, IL 60610-7224
(800) 826-3632
www.dbsalliance.org

Depression and Related Affective Disorders Association
2330 W. Joppa Road, Suite 100
Lutherville, MD 21093
(410) 583-2919
www.drada.org

Families and Advocates Partnership for Education
PACER Center
8161 Normandale Boulevard
Minneapolis, MN 55437-1044
(952) 838-9000
www.fape.org

Federation of Families for Children's Mental Health
1101 King Street, Suite 420
Alexandria, VA 22314
(703) 684-7710
www.ffcmh.org

Food and Drug Administration
5600 Fishers Lane
Rockville, MD 20857
(888) 463-6332
www.fda.gov

Jed Foundation
583 Broadway, Suite 8B
New York, NY 10012
(212) 647-7544
www.jedfoundation.org

National Alliance for Research on Schizophrenia and Depression
60 Cutter Mill Road, Suite 404
Great Neck, NY 11021
(800) 829-8289
www.narsad.org

National Alliance for the Mentally Ill
Colonial Place Three
2107 Wilson Boulevard, Suite 300
Arlington, VA 22201-3042
(800) 950-6264
www.nami.org

National Dissemination Center for Children with Disabilities
P.O. Box 1492
Washington, DC 20013
(800) 695-0285
www.nichcy.org

National Hopeline Network
Kristin Brooks Hope Center
2001 N. Beauregard Street, 12th Floor
Alexandria, VA 22311
(800) 784-2433
www.hopeline.com

National Institute of Mental Health
Office of Communications
6001 Executive Boulevard, Room 8184, MSC 9663
Bethesda, MD 20892-9663
(866) 615-6464
www.nimh.nih.gov

National Mental Health Association
2001 N. Beauregard Street, 12th Floor
Alexandria, VA 22311
(800) 969-6642
www.nmha.org

National Mental Health Information Center
Substance Abuse and Mental Health Services Administration
P.O. Box 42557
Washington, DC 20015
(800) 789-2647
www.mentalhealth.org

Suicide Awareness Voices of Education
9001 E. Bloomington Freeway, Suite 150
Bloomington, MN 55420
(952) 946-7998
www.save.org

## Books

American Medical Association. *American Medical Association Essential Guide to Depression.* New York: Pocket Books, 1998.

Birmaher, Boris. *New Hope for Children and Teens With Bipolar Disorder.* New York: Three Rivers Press, 2004.

Empfield, Maureen, and Nicholas Bakalar. *Understanding Teenage Depression: A Guide to Diagnosis, Treatment, and Management.* New York: Owl Books, 2001.

Fassler, David G., and Lynne S. Dumas. *"Help Me, I'm Sad": Recognizing, Treating, and Preventing Childhood and Adolescent Depression.* New York: Viking, 1997.

Fristad, Mary A., and Jill S. Goldberg Arnold. *Raising a Moody Child: How to Cope With Depression and Bipolar Disorder.* New York: Guilford Press, 2004.

Greene, Ross W. *The Explosive Child: A New Approach for Understanding and Parenting Easily Frustrated, Chronically Inflexible Children.* New York: Quill, 2001.

Ingersoll, Barbara D., and Sam Goldstein. *Lonely, Sad and Angry: A Parent's Guide to Depression in Children and Adolescents.* New York: Doubleday, 1995.

Jamison, Kay Redfield. *Night Falls Fast: Understanding Suicide.* New York: Alfred A. Knopf, 1999.

Jamison, Kay Redfield. *Touched With Fire: Manic-Depressive Illness and the Artistic Temperament.* New York: Simon and Schuster, 1993.

Kaufman, Miriam. *Overcoming Teen Depression: A Guide for Parents.* Buffalo, NY: Firefly Books, 2001.

Lederman, Judith, and Candida Fink. *The Ups and Downs of Raising a Bipolar Child: A Survival Guide for Parents.* New York: Fireside, 2003.

Mondimore, Francis Mark. *Adolescent Depression: A Guide for Parents.* Baltimore: Johns Hopkins University Press, 2002.

Oster, Gerald D., and Sarah S. Montgomery. *Helping Your Depressed Teenager: A Guide for Parents and Caregivers.* New York: John Wiley and Sons, 1995.

Papolos, Demitri, and Janice Papolos. *The Bipolar Child: The Definitive and Reassuring Guide to Childhood's Most Misunderstood Disorder* (rev. ed.). New York: Broadway Books, 2002.

Raeburn, Paul. *Acquainted With the Night: A Parent's Quest to Understand Depression and Bipolar Disorder in His Children.* New York: Broadway Books, 2004.

Rosenthal, Norman E. *Winter Blues: Seasonal Affective Disorder—What It Is and How to Overcome It* (rev. ed.). New York: Guilford Press, 1998.

Seligman, Martin E. P., with Karen Reivich, Lisa Jaycox, and Jane Gillham. *The Optimistic Child: A Proven Program to Safeguard Children Against Depression and Build Lifelong Resilience.* New York: Houghton Mifflin, 1995.

Thase, Michael E., and Susan S. Lang. *Beating the Blues: New Approaches to Overcoming Dysthymia and Chronic Mild Depression.* New York: Oxford University Press, 2004.

Waltz, Mitzi. *Bipolar Disorders: A Guide to Helping Children and Adolescents.* Sebastopol, CA: O'Reilly, 2000.

Wilens, Timothy E. *Straight Talk About Psychiatric Medications for Kids.* New York: Guilford Press, 2004.

## Websites

Depression-Screening.org, National Mental Health Association, www.depression screening.org

Family Guide to Keeping Youth Mentally Healthy and Drug Free, Substance Abuse and Mental Health Services Administration, www.family.samhsa.gov

# Resources for Adolescents

## Books

Cobain, Bev. *When Nothing Matters Anymore: A Survival Guide for Depressed Teens.* Minneapolis: Free Spirit, 1998.

Irwin, Cait. *Conquering the Beast Within: How I Fought Depression and Won . . . and How You Can, Too.* New York: Three Rivers Press, 1999.

## Websites

MindZone, Annenberg Foundation Trust at Sunnylands with the Annenberg Public Policy Center of the University of Pennsylvania, www.fhidc.com/annenberg/copecaredeal

TeensHealth, Nemours Foundation, www.teenshealth.org

# Resources for Related Problems

## Anxiety disorders

### *Book*

Foa, Edna B., and Linda Wasmer Andrews. *If Your Adolescent Has an Anxiety Disorder: An Essential Resource for Parents.* New York: Oxford University Press with the Annenberg Foundation Trust at Sunnylands and the Annenberg Public Policy Center at the University of Pennsylvania, forthcoming 2006.

### *Website*

Anxiety Disorders Association of America, (240) 485-1001, www.adaa.org

## Attention-deficit hyperactivity disorder

Attention-deficit Disorder Association, (484) 945-2101, www.add.org

Children and Adults with Attention-Deficit/Hyperactivity Disorder, (800) 233-4050, www.help4adhd.org

## Eating disorders

### *Book*

Walsh, B. Timothy, and V. L. Cameron. *If Your Adolescent Has an Eating Disorder: An Essential Resource for Parents.* New York: Oxford University Press with the Annenberg Foundation Trust at Sunnylands and the Annenberg Public Policy Center at the University of Pennsylvania, forthcoming 2005.

## *Websites*

National Association of Anorexia Nervosa and Associated Disorders, (847) 831-3438, www.anad.org

National Eating Disorders Association, (206) 382-3587, www.nationaleating disorders.org

## Learning disorders

International Dyslexia Association, (410) 296-0232, www.interdys.org

LD OnLine, www.ldonline.org

Learning Disabilities Association of America, (412) 341-1515, www.ldaamerica.org

National Center for Learning Disabilities, (888) 575-7373, www.ld.org

## Substance abuse

Alcoholics Anonymous, (212) 870-3400 (check your phone book for a local number), www.aa.org

American Council for Drug Education, (800) 488-3784, www.acde.org

Leadership to Keep Children Alcohol Free, (301) 654-6740, www.alcohol freechildren.org

Narcotics Anonymous, (818) 773-9999, www.na.org

National Council on Alcoholism and Drug Dependence, (800) 622-2255, www.ncadd.org

National Institute on Alcohol Abuse and Alcoholism, (301) 443–3860, www.niaaa.nih.gov

National Institute on Drug Abuse, (301) 443-1124, www.drug abuse.gov

National Youth Anti-Drug Media Campaign, (800) 666-3332, www.mediacampaign.org

Partnership for a Drug-Free America, (212) 922-1560, www.drug freeamerica.com

Substance Abuse and Mental Health Services Administration, (800) 662-4357, www.samhsa.gov

# Bibliography

American Psychiatric Association. *Diagnostic and Statistical Manual of Mental Disorders* (4th ed., text revision). Washington, DC: American Psychiatric Association, 2000.

Andersen, Margot, Jane Boyd Kubisak, Ruth Field, and Steven Vogelstein. *Understanding and Educating Children and Adolescents With Bipolar Disorder: A Guide for Educators.* Northfield, IL: Josselyn Center, 2003.

Bazelon Center for Mental Health Law. *Avoiding Cruel Choices: A Guide for Policymakers and Family Organizations on Medicaid's Role in Preventing Custody Relinquishment.* Washington, DC: Bazelon Center for Mental Health Law, 2002.

Bazelon Center for Mental Health Law. *Suspending Disbelief: Moving Beyond Punishment to Promote Effective Interventions for Children With Mental or Emotional Disorders.* Washington, DC: Bazelon Center for Mental Health Law, 2003.

Bazelon Center for Mental Health Law. *Teaming Up: Using the IDEA and Medicaid to Secure Comprehensive Mental Health Services for Children and Youth.* Washington, DC: Bazelon Center for Mental Health Law, 2003.

Evans, Dwight L., Edna B. Foa, Raquel E. Gur, Herbert Hendin, Charles P. O'Brien, Martin E. P. Seligman, and B. Timothy Walsh. *Treating and Preventing Adolescent Mental Health Disorders: What We Know and What We Don't Know.* New York: Oxford University Press with the Annenberg Foundation Trust at Sunnylands and the Annenberg Public Policy Center at the University of Pennsylvania, 2005.

Findling, Robert L., Robert A. Kowatch, and Robert M. Post. *Pediatric Bipolar Disorder: A Handbook for Clinicians.* London: Martin Dunitz, 2003.

Geller, Barbara, and Melissa P. DelBello (Eds.). *Bipolar Disorder in Childhood and Early Adolescence.* New York: Guilford Press, 2003.

Shaffer, David, and Bruce D. Waslick (Eds.). *The Many Faces of Depression in Children and Adolescents.* Washington, DC: American Psychiatric Publishing, 2002.

U.S. General Accounting Office. *Child Welfare and Juvenile Justice: Federal Agencies Could Play a Stronger Role in Helping States Reduce the Number of Children Placed Solely to Obtain Mental Health Services* (GAO-03-397). Washington, DC: U.S. General Accounting Office, 2003.

U.S. Public Health Service. *Report of the Surgeon General's Conference on Children's Mental Health: A National Action Agenda.* Washington, DC: Department of Health and Human Services, 2000.

# Index

# About the Authors

**Dwight L. Evans**, M.D. is the Ruth Meltzer Professor and Chairman of the Department of Psychiatry and Professor of Psychiatry, Medicine and Neuroscience at the University of Pennsylvania School of Medicine in Philadelphia. He was chair of the Adolescent Mental Health Initiative's formal Commission on Depression and Bipolar Disorder, from which this book draws much of its scientific information. Dr. Evans has received numerous awards including The Beck Award for excellence in suicidology from the American Foundation for Suicide Prevention and the Mood Disorders Research Award for major contributions to the understanding and treatment of mood disorders from the American College of Psychiatrists.

**Linda Wasmer Andrews** is a freelance science writer based in Albuquerque, New Mexico. She is the author of nine books, including *Emotional Intelligence* (for young readers), and a regular contributor to *Self* magazine.